THE INTERESTS OF PHARMACISTS

THE INTERESTS OF PHARMACISTS

Milton Schwebel

Submitted in partial fulfillment of the requirements
for the degree of Doctor of Philosophy
in the Faculty of Philosophy
Columbia University

KING'S CROWN PRESS
Columbia University, New York   1951

TO MY MOTHER AND FATHER

Copyright 1951 by Milton Schwebel
King's Crown Press is an imprint established by Columbia University Press
for the purpose of making certain scholarly material available at minimum cost.
Toward that end, the publishers have used standardized formats incorporating every reasonable economy
that does not interfere with legibility. The author has assumed complete responsibility
for editorial style and for proofreading.

Published in Great Britain, Canada and India, by Geoffrey Cumberlege, Oxford University Press
London, Toronto, and Bombay
Manufactured in the United States of America

Lithoprinted in U.S.A.
EDWARDS BROTHERS, INC.
ANN ARBOR, MICHIGAN
1951

Foreword

FOR twenty-five years psychologists, counselors, and personnel men have used interest inventories in diagnosing interests and in estimating prospects of success and satisfaction in various fields of work. One of their fundamental assumptions has been that men and women who are interested in their work and who have interests like those of others in their vocation will find satisfaction in their work. Interest inventories have therefore become a principal tool of counselors and personnel workers, and of these Strong's Vocational Interest Blank is one of the most carefully developed and widely used.

The foundation of Strong's work was the finding that persons successfully engaged in an occupation have interests which differentiate them from men or women in other occupations. Despite a quarter century of fruitful research, however, two important questions have been insufficiently explored by Strong and other interest researchers. These are, first, the relationship between inventoried interest and work satisfaction (as distinguished from success or continued employment), and secondly, the differentiation of specialties within an occupation.

In the research reported in this monograph, Dr. Schwebel has added significantly to our knowledge of both these topics. Selecting pharmacists as the subjects of his study, he has worked with an occupational group which has recently been submitting itself to much self-study because of the dissatisfaction which is widespread among pharmacists and which has created recruiting problems for that profession. Developing several scoring scales, using both Strong's method and methods of his own which contrast satisfied with dissatisfied members of the occupation and members of one specialty (apothecaries) with members of another specialty (retail business), Dr. Schwebel has shown that the interests of most prescription and research pharmacists are not clearly different from those of most retail druggists, he has confirmed the validity of Strong's men-in-general reference point in interest scale construction; and he has demonstrated the need for, and value of, adding a satisfaction criterion to the occupational success and stability criteria used by Strong in selecting criterion groups. In addition to these theoretical and technical contributions, Dr. Schwebel has made available a new scoring key for Strong's Vocational Interest Blank, thereby making that widely used test useful also for counseling and selecting potential pharmacists.

FOREWORD

These contributions should be of interest to vocational counselors and to personnel workers using interest inventories in counseling individuals or in selecting employees, to industrial relations specialists interested in problems of work and job satisfaction, and especially to personnel psychologists who are engaged in test construction and evaluation.

Donald E. Super

Teachers College, Columbia University
January 2, 1951

Acknowledgments

THE amount of work in the study was out of proportion to the size of this volume, and the help of many persons made its completion possible. Thanks are gratefully extended to the following:

The sponsors of the study for their invaluable aid, often given at their own inconvenience via long-distance correspondence: Dr. Irving Lorge and Dr. Laurance F. Shaffer, of Teachers College, Columbia University, and especially Dr. Donald E. Super for the respect for science that he fostered, for his kindness and understanding;

The endorsers of the investigation, Dean Charles W. Ballard, College of Pharmacy, Columbia University: Dean A. B. Lemon, School of Pharmacy, University of Buffalo; Dean Francis J. O'Brien, Albany College of Pharmacy, Union University; Dr. Curt P. Wimmer, Public Relations Director, New York State Pharmaceutical Association;

The hundreds of pharmacists in New York State and Connecticut who gave generously of their time to provide the data of the study, especially the many pharmacists in Utica, New York, and the members of the New Haven Druggists Association who sponsored his trip to New Haven and patiently devoted most of one meeting to filling in questionnaires;

Dr. Harry D. Kitson, of Teachers College, Columbia University for encouragement and suggestions prior to, and during, the investigation; Dr. Edward K. Strong Jr., of the Vocational Interest Research Project, Stanford University, for much encouraging help and special scoring arrangements[1];Dr. Robert Hoppock, New York University, now the writer's department chairman and colleague, for permission to use his Job Satisfaction Blank No. 1; Dr. Robert L. Thorndike, of Teachers College, Columbia University; Dr. Edward C. Elliott, Director of the Pharmaceutical Survey of the American Council of Education, and Dr. H. H. Remmers, Director of the Survey's Student Personnel Studies;

---

1. Both IBM and hand-scoring keys for the new Vocational Interest Scale for Pharmacists are available through Stanford University Press, Stanford University, California. Engineers Northwest, Minneapolis 1, Minnesota, now scores the Hankes answer sheet for the Strong Blank for pharmacy interest.

Dr. Dorothy M. Clendenen, of the University of California; Dean H. G. Hewitt, of the College of Pharmacy, University of Connecticut; and Dean H. C. Newton, of the Massachusetts College of Pharmacy; the many who volunteered their time for tedious clerical work: friends on the Mohawk College Faculty in Utica; and Sara and Joseph Davison; Rosalind Ivanhoe; A. A. Gaies; Tobie and Herman Kessler;

The writer's sons, one of whom patiently tolerated frequent interference with playtime plans, and the other of whom considerately delayed his arrival until a propitious time; and most of all to the writer's wife who at all stages of the study helped maintain research interest and satisfaction.

Milton Schwebel

New York University
December 20, 1950

Contents

Foreword by Donald E. Super	v
I. THE PROBLEM	1
II. CONCEPTS OF JOB SATISFACTION	10
III. DESIGN OF THE STUDY	13
IV. DIFFERENTIATING CHARACTERISTICS OF THE SATISFIED AND DISSATISFIED	17
V. CONSTRUCTION OF THREE PHARMACY INTEREST SCALES	32
VI. EFFECTIVENESS OF THE SCALES	39
VII. INTERRELATIONSHIP AND EVALUATION OF SCALES	58
VIII. SUMMARY AND CONCLUSIONS	66
APPENDIX	71
BIBLIOGRAPHY	75
INDEX	81

Tables

1. Size of Sample 15
2. Nondifferentiating Characteristics of 333 Satisfied and 117 Dissatisfied Pharmacists 19
3. Differences in Percentages of Satisfied and Dissatisfied Pharmacists for Various Age Groups 20
4. Differentiating Characteristics of 333 Satisfied and 117 Dissatisfied Pharmacists 21
5. Satisfaction in Apothecary and Business Pharmacist Groups 22
6. Age Distribution of 50 Least and 50 Most Satisfied Pharmacists.............................. 24
7. Years in Pharmacy of 50 Least and 50 Most Satisfied Pharmacists......................... 25
8. Percentage of Time Spent on Prescription work of Satisfied and Dissatisfied Pharmacists in Standardization Group and Extreme Subgroups 26
9. Occupation in Pharmacy of 50 Least and 50 Most Satisfied Pharmacists 27
10. Composition of the Three New Pharmacy Scales .. 36
11. Scores and Letter Grades for Three Pharmacy Scales 37
12. Percentage of Norm Group in Each Scoring Category on Three Pharmacy Scales 38
13. Difference in Mean Standard Scores of 105 Validation Group Pharmacists on Pharmacy Scales and 424 Standardization Group Pharmacists on Six Non-Pharmacy Scales. 43
14. Percentage of Pharmacists with A, B, and C Grades on Three Pharmacy and Six Non-Pharmacy Scales. 45
15. Mean Standard Scores of 105 Validation Group Pharmacists and 52 Medical College Upperclassmen on Pharmacy Scales 46

16. Differences in Mean Standard Scores of 52 Medical Upperclassmen on Physician and on Three Pharmacy Scales 47
17. Letter Grades of 52 Medical Upperclassmen on Physician and Pharmacy Scales 47
18. Standard Scores of 152 Apothecary and 135 Business Satisfied Pharmacists on Six Non-Pharmacy Scales 48
19. Difference in Mean Standard Scores of 71 Satisfied Pharmacists on S-D Scale and Other Pharmacy Scales 50
20. Difference between 71 Satisfied and 32 Dissatisfied Validation-Group Pharmacists on Three Pharmacy Scales 51
21. Difference between 71 Satisfied and 32 Dissatisfied Validation-Group in Percentage of A and of Combined A and B+ Letter Grades 52
22. Comparison of 313 Satisfied and 111 Dissatisfied Standardization-Group on Six Non-Pharmacy Scales 53
23. Difference in Mean Standard Score of 49 Apothecary Pharmacists on A-B and Other Pharmacy Scales .. 54
24. Difference between Apothecary and Business Pharmacists on Three Pharmacy Scales 55
25. Difference between 49 Apothecary and 48 Business Pharmacists in Percentages of A, and of Combined A and B+ Letter Grades 56
26. Intercorrelations of Scores of 105 Validation-Group Pharmacists on Three Pharmacy Scales 58
27. Intercorrelations of Scores of 71 Validation-Group Pharmacists on Three Pharmacy Scales 59
28. Odd-Even Half-Scale Correlations of Scores of 105 Validation-Group Pharmacists within and between Three Pharmacy Scales 60
29. Correlations of Index of Satisfaction on Pharmacy Satisfaction Scale and of Standard Score on Three Pharmacy Interest Scales, for 103 Validation-Group Pharmacists. 61

I The Problem

THE rapid growth of clinical and vocational psychology during the past two decades indicates the great interest increasingly being shown in the adjustment of the individual in society. No matter what differences in interpretation may exist concerning the causal factors in this trend, the fact that it has occurred and that it continues cannot be gainsaid. As Wolfle (80) stated in his annual report to the American Psychological Association for 1948, the increasing influence of the psychologist obligates him to evaluate the efficacy of the tools and techniques he employs, and to create new instruments for use in service to the community.

In their efforts to aid student and worker in the choice of an occupational milieu compatible with their personalities, psychologists have devised and improved the technique of the interest inventory. They have gone beyond the simple score or "I.Q." stage and are concerned with the clinical implications and interpretations of interest patterns (9). Whether judged in terms of their reliability and validity, or in terms of the extensiveness of their use, the interest inventories most commonly used today have achieved a high degree of success. They have increased the effectiveness of psychological measurement in the prediction of vocational success, a significant contribution to vocational guidance. Studies that have neglected motivational factors, such as vocational interests, have not been effective in making such predictions (39, 40, 73). There are still few studies which furnish clear-cut evidence of the validity of the interest inventory in forecasting vocational success, but Strong's work with life insurance salesmen (56, 63) and with Stanford University seniors (61, 63) suggests that it is an indispensable tool for vocational prediction.

Reviews of the literature indicate that interest measurement (6, 17, 63) has been a prolific area of research, hence the significant advances that have been made. Continued investigation is necessary for further refinements of the technique. This research is an attempt to examine certain problems that may be crucial to the subsequent development of interest inventories.

This study utilizes only one interest measure, the Strong Vocational Interest Blank for Men. One of the most widely used measures, it has been described as long being "the outstanding device of its kind" (6). Strong[1] has found that men engaged in a particular occupation can be differentiated from men in other occupations by their pattern of likes and dislikes. The large number of items in the bank, the variety of human activities included, and the opportunity for the examinee to make one of three different responses, make it possible to differentiate the interest patterns of the various occupations in so far as perceptible differences exist. It is then a simple matter to discover with which occupational scales or patterns of interests any individual's interests most nearly agree. It is assumed that he is most likely to find congenial those occupations with which the agreement of likes and dislikes is substantial.

Strong writes in his manual that "if a man likes to do the things which men like who are successful in a given occupation and dislikes to do the things which these same men dislike to do, he will feel at home in that occupational environment. Seemingly, also, he should be more effective there than somewhere else because he would be engaged, in the main, in work he liked." Strong has succeeded in validating these assumptions for groups in a follow-up study of Stanford seniors[2]. The success he has achieved in validating his hypothesis and the exceptions he has found within the groups raise a number of questions. Those which follow are the problems with which this study is concerned:

1. The responses of an individual on the Vocational Interest Blank are compared with those of "successful" men in an occupation. The criterion of success usually used in selecting the criterion group is that its members shall be continuing in an occupation in which they have been engaged for at least three years. If it is possible to measure the agreement of the examinee's interests with those of men engaged in the occupation for at least three years, <u>is it also</u> possible to measure the agreement of his interests with those of men engaged in the occupation for three years who are also "satisfied" with that occupation? With the criterion of success that Strong has used, the interest pattern of an occupational group has pre-

---

1. Except when otherwise indicated, subsequent references to Strong are to item 63 in the Bibliography.
2. For further discussion of validation, see <u>infra</u>.

THE PROBLEM 3

sumably been contaminated by the likes and dislikes of its dissatisfied members. <u>By excluding them from the weighting and standardization groups, can an interest scale be developed which will differentiate the satisfied from the dissatisfied persons in this occupation</u>?

Strong has pointed out that interest inventories discriminate poorly or not at all between successful and unsuccessful groups within some occupations, for example teaching, although they perform better in differentiating comparable groups of life insurance salesmen. He suggests that achievement may be a poor criterion of the validity of an interest inventory because men may have the same interest in "the kinds of things which are handled" in a given occupation, yet have varying abilities to manipulate these tools (mechanical, social, intellectual). Either the interests of the two are not different or, he adds, our methods are still inadequate to differentiate them. As interest inventories have not proven very successful in predicting quantitatively evaluated achievement, it has been generally assumed that they suggest areas of probable satisfaction. Strong has written that "interests indicate satisfaction," and in the lengthier quotation above he asserts that if an individual has interests characteristic of those successful in it, "he will feel at home in that occupational environment." If predicting satisfaction in an occupation is a primary objective of interest measurement, then it seems advisable to ascertain whether or not the introduction of "satisfaction" into the criterion in addition to "success" (three years in the occupation) would make for better prediction. In a review of Strong's book, Super (69) has written: "In spite of widespread acceptance of the hypothesis concerning the significance of vocational interests for personal and vocational adjustment, surprisingly little research has been done in the prediction of satisfaction." Referring then to several studies on the relation between satisfaction and interest, he adds: "Findings such as these would seem to warrant discussion and further research."

2. An occupational scale is constructed by contrasting the percentage of like, indifferent, or dislike responses of the members of the occupation to each of the 400 items on the blank, with the comparable responses of the "men-in-general" group, and by weighting each of the 1200 possible responses in accordance with the difference between the two groups. The greater the difference between the two in response to an item, the heavier is the weight assigned that item on the occupation's scoring scale. The scale simply indicates the degree

to which men in a specific occupation differ in their interests from men-in-general (a fair representation of business and professional men earning $2500 and over a year). Several recent studies, discussed below, have suggested that the use of a point of reference other than men-in-general for contrast with the occupational group being studied yields a sharper delineation of the members of the occupation in terms of their interests. This then is a second question with which this study is concerned: if the satisfied members of an occupation can be differentiated by their interests from the dissatisfied, can this be done more effectively by constructing a scale in which the satisfied are contrasted with the dissatisfied, than by contrasting the satisfied with the men-in-general? <u>Will the dissatisfied members of an occupation serve as a better point of reference than a group of men-in-general in constructing an interest-measuring device for the differentiation of the satisfied?</u>

3. It was decided to use members of the pharmacy profession as subjects to test the hypotheses implied in the two questions discussed above. A new interest scale had first to be developed, for pharmacy was one of the few major professions that had none. This raised an additional question which, <u>a priori</u>, seemed likely to be answered affirmatively: <u>Do the interests of pharmacists form a pattern distinguishable from those of other occupations?</u>

4. Perhaps the effectiveness of interest inventories can be improved by reexamining not merely the techniques of measurement but also the definitions of the occupations that are studied. With its dual function as an applied science and as a business, pharmacy is peculiarly suited to the investigation of this problem. This study will seek to answer a fourth question: <u>Can the "business" pharmacists who devote less than 25 per cent of their time to prescription work or research be differentiated by their interests from the "apothecary" pharmacists who devote more than 25 per cent of their time to the scientific activities of the profession?</u>

THE PROBLEM

INFERENCES FROM RELEVANT STUDIES

The hypotheses of this study are restated below in positive form, each followed by discussion of the relevant research reported in the literature of the past decade.

1. By making satisfaction in pharmacy, as well as three-year membership in the occupation, a criterion in selecting a norm group for the construction of an interest scale, it will be possible to differentiate satisfied pharmacists from both non-pharmacists and dissatisfied pharmacists.

In a study of 100 non-college adults, 76 men and 24 women, Sarbin and Anderson (46) tested the hypothesis that adults dissatisfied with their current occupations do not have a primary interest pattern in the occupational interest group in which their present occupation is located; that is, they do not have a majority or plurality of A and B+ scores on the Strong Vocational Interest Blank in the group of occupations in which their current occupation belongs; either they have no A or B+ scores or those that they have are in occupational groups that do not include their own occupation. They found that 82 per cent of the males and 58 per cent of the females "who complain of occupational dissatisfaction show no primary pattern of interest in the group of occupations which embraces their present occupation." They concluded that dissatisfaction with the current occupation was associated with lack of primary interest in it.

This would suggest that the exclusion of the occupationally dissatisfied from the groups used in constructing a scale would make for greater homogeneity of interest, and would consequently make for a more effective measuring device.

In measuring the interests of Marine Corps women reservists Hahn and Williams (22), using the Kuder Preference Record, found that three groups of clerical workers (stenographers, clerk-typists, and general clerks) satisfied with their jobs had interest profiles which were much more clearly differentiated from the interest patterns of the total standardization groups of almost eight hundred women than subsamples containing a large proportion of individuals disinterested in, or dissatisfied with, their current occupations. They concluded that the norming groups for interest inventories should be composed only of those who are satisfied with their jobs.

The relationship between job satisfaction and interests has been given relatively little attention, as Darley (10) has recently written. He emphasizes the importance of research "directed toward the interests of defined maladjusted groups of workers and students, in an effort to determine the part played by measured interests in creating or alleviating occupational and educational dissatisfaction or failure." Here we are more concerned with development of techniques for the differentiation of the interests of the satisfied and the dissatisfied pharmacists, but it is expected that this research will cast some light upon the relationship between interests and occupational maladjustment and that it will suggest hypotheses for further investigation.

2. The differentiation of satisfied pharmacists from both non-pharmacists and dissatisfied pharmacists can be best achieved by substituting the dissatisfied pharmacists for the men-in-general group as the point of reference.

Several studies suggest the advantages of using a point of reference other than the composite men-in-general group. In developing the occupational-level scale Strong compared the interests of unskilled men with those of business and professional men earning $2500 and more, at a time when only about one seventh of American families were in that income group.

By contrasting the interests of one group of engineering students with those of four other groups, Estes and Horn (13) constructed five independent scales for the following branches of engineering: civil, electrical, chemical, industrial, and mechanical. They succeeded in differentiating the interests of students in the various engineering curricula to the extent that only 11 per cent of the men not enrolled in the curriculum for which they were scored earned a letter rating of A, and 43.5 per cent earned C, as compared with 75.5 per cent A and three per cent C for those enrolled in the curriculum for which they were scored. This successful differentiation was made on subgroups of the original criterion group and not on new cross-validation groups.

In a study by Ryan and Johnson (45) the subjects were workers employed in two different occupations rather than students. In seeking to differentiate between the "good" and "poor" workers in each of these occupations (business machine salesmen and servicemen) they found that the ability-group keys in which the superior are contrasted with the inferior were better than the traditional occupational scoring keys in which all of the men in the occupation (good and poor) are contrasted with men-in-general. The difference in interest scores on the ability-group keys between the good and the poor worker was significant for the norm group, but not for the validation group. The authors conclude that their results "permit us to suggest that the

THE PROBLEM

ability-group method of weighting items on the Strong Vocational Interest Blank may sometimes be more useful than the current methods of weighting." This method "also showed a definite promise of distinguishing between good and poor men even within the control groups which had not been used in the determination of weights. This differentiation was possible even though the employees we studied were already carefully selected according to traditional methods."

When one of the scales for the Strong Blank is constructed for any occupation, as for example engineering, the interests common to engineers and men-in-general are excluded, and the unique interests are used to establish weights for scoring. What Estes and Horn did, as Strong pointed out, was to cancel out the interests which are common to engineers, and to base their five new scales on interests specific to the subgroups, on interests, that is, that civil engineers have but that other engineers do not have. These scales should be useful when a student knows he wants the general field of engineering but is not sure in which area he wishes to specialize. Are they equally effective in differentiating the interests of engineers from those of non-engineers? This is a significant question, for if it is answered negatively, perhaps we will find that a scale constructed by contrasting satisfied and dissatisfied pharmacists will differentiate the two successfully but will not differentiate pharmacists from non-pharmacists. A tentative answer is provided in the study by Ryan and Johnson. The sales ability key was constructed by contrasting good and poor salesmen. No other workers were involved in determining the weights. Yet this scale which differentiated good from poor salesmen clearly differentiated salesmen from non-salesmen.

3. The interests of pharmacists are distinguishable from those of other occupational groups.

Any occupation might have been used to investigate the first two hypotheses, but few were as well suited to the fourth (discussed below) as pharmacy. This, however, was only one reason for the selection of pharmacy. The necessity of separating the interest blanks into a satisfied and a dissatisfied group precluded the possibility of using old blanks for this study without further contact with the subjects. Since such contact was necessary it was deemed wise to construct entirely new scales. The selection of pharmacy seemed logical since the pharmacy profession had been experiencing developmental difficulties and was at the time of this research having a thorough analysis of its status made under the sponsorship of the American Council on Education. This investigation, a report of which has been published (82), sought particularly to clarify the objectives of pharmaceutical education in the light of the present-day practices and the future needs of pharmacy. After devoting more than two years to the tasks of "assembling, organizing and interpreting the essential facts relating to American pharmacy" the Committee on the Pharmaceutical Survey recommended a number of programs of action, the goal of which "is the setting up and maintenance of standards that will justify the recognition of pharmacy as a high-level profession in every section of the country." In the chapter on "Student Selection, Guidance, and Testing," the recommendation is made that pharmaceutical training institutions utilize tests in the selection of students and that the American Association of Colleges of Pharmacy take steps for the development and validation of such tests. It was thought that this study could both contribute to our knowledge of interest measurement and provide counselors and admissions officers with a helpful tool.

There seemed no doubt that the interests of pharmacists would form a pattern different from that of other occupational groups. Some occupations, however, are so closely related to each other that little differentiation between them is possible. The physicist scale, for example, is no longer published because it correlates .93 with that for chemist and .91 with that for mathematician. These occupational groups had too much in common with each other when contrasted with the men-in-general to be clearly differentiated from each other. The high correlation in itself is not evidence of error in test construction, but rather of agreement in interest of the members of these two professions. Where greater differentiation is desired, the techniques of contrasting the interests of the two and finding their unique interests must be used. It seemed unlikely that pharmacy, with a combination of applied science and salesmanship unmatched by any other field for which Strong's Blank can be scored, would be so close to any other occupations in the constellation of occupational interests as to make it undifferentiable.

4. Pharmacy consists of two separate occupational groups, "apothecary" and "businessman," whose interest patterns are distinguishable.

If any close relationship existed between pharmacists and members of other occupational groups, it was believed that these pharmacists would be part of a subgroup of their profession, i.e., apothecaries or businessmen. It seemed conceivable that the interests of apothecary pharmacists might be positively

THE PROBLEM

correlated with those of chemists, physicians, and dentists, and the interests of business pharmacists with those of life insurance salesmen, real estate salesmen, sales managers, and office men. If the interests of these two subgroups are different, as their functions in pharmacy are different, verification of this fact may be of significance in the selection, training, and placement of pharmacists. Perhaps as a consequence the present definition of pharmacy in the <u>Dictionary of Occupational Titles</u>[3], with only slight revision would be assigned to the apothecary pharmacist, and another one to the business pharmacist. In view of the high percentage of sales work involved in pharmacy today, this definition appears to be unrealistic. The opinion of even the older workers in pharmacy tends to bear this out. Noall (42) reports that experienced pharmacists consider salesmanship, accuracy, honesty, manual dexterity, and cleanliness as the qualities which contribute toward success in their profession.

The technique used with success by Estes and Horn in differentiating the various branches of engineering by contrasting their interests without intermediation of a men-in-general group, and the similar experience of Ryan and Johnson with the good and poor salesmen and servicemen, was selected for use in constructing the Apothecary vs. Business Pharmacist Interest Scale, in an attempt to differentiate the interests of the two. If this scale differentiates the apothecary and business members of a validation group of pharmacists it can be concluded that the differences of interest upon which the weights are based are unique interests peculiar to apothecaries and business pharmacists.

---

3. PHARMACIST: apothecary; druggist; registered pharmacist (profess. & kin.) 0-25.10 Compounds and dispenses medicines and preparations as directed by prescriptions prepared by licensed PHYSICIANS (med. ser.) and DENTISTS (med. ser.); performs various assays and tests to determine identity, purity and strength of drugs; preserves drugs, medicines, biologicals, or chemicals; maintains stock of drugs, chemicals, and other pharmaceutical supplies.

II   Concepts of Job Satisfaction

A REVIEW of the literature on job satisfaction (24, 25, 27, 28, 29, 30, 31) indicates that one of the greatest difficulties in research in this field is in defining the concept of satisfaction. Its meaning has varied with the techniques used in the investigation, the occupation studied, and whether the data were to be used in attacking the problem of industrial absenteeism or surveying the extent and nature of dissatisfaction in a profession such as teaching.

This is not a study of job satisfaction. It does not propose to clarify the concept of worker morale. Rather it is an attempt to ascertain the value of basing interest inventories only on those who consider themselves satisfied, and of comparing them with those who consider themselves dissatisfied. It makes no pretense at probing the deeper layers of personality to discover if the origin of dissatisfaction predates vocational life, or to differentiate between those who are dissatisfied only under certain conditions and those who appear to be dissatisfied under any occupational conditions. That such a difference exists is suggested by the findings of Super (67) in a study of the interest patterns of four groups of hobbyists. When compared with stamp collectors, model engineers, and photographers, amateur musicians tended to be more dissatisfied with their jobs and to favor their hobby as compared with their vocation in disproportionate numbers. Only 56 per cent of the musicians were socially adjusted (as judged by the satisfying social contacts they had) as compared with 92, 88, and 86 per cent respectively for the other three groups of hobbyists. Super believes this indicates that the vocational dissatisfaction of the musicians is only one aspect of general maladjustment, while that of the other groups is localized dissatisfaction with their work.

In this study, these two types (general maladjustment and localized job dissatisfaction) have not been differentiated. No steps were taken to discover what forces were at work in the private life of the individual that might have produced low morale, nor what mishaps might have befallen the subject and made him disgruntled momentarily before filling out the forms. That such factors are influential cannot be denied; they have caused some progressive industrial concerns to introduce employee counseling services to deal with the personal problems that lead to dissatisfaction (11, 19). In research these

CONCEPTS OF JOB SATISFACTION

conditions are difficult to control. Whereas the skilled interviewer can frequently determine whether an attitude of a worker toward his occupation is stable or only the temporary effect of some unusual incident, the interview technique, which has experimental imperfections of its own, can rarely be used when data must be obtained from large numbers of persons.

For this study, as for many others whose objective is not definitive conclusions on the nature of job attitudes, a pragmatic definition like Hoppock's (25) is a satisfactory guide: job satisfaction is "any combination of psychological, physiological, or environmental circumstances that causes a person truthfully to say 'I am satisfied with my job.'" Hand (23) describes it as "the whole matrix of job factors that make a person like his work situation and be willing to head for it without distaste at the beginning of his workday." Our information comes precisely in this form. The pharmacist indicates on the satisfaction scale whether he is glad or sorry he is a pharmacist; the degree to which he likes being a pharmacist (e.g., "I hate it."); his evaluation of his attitude toward pharmacy as compared with other people's attitude toward their work; how much of the time he feels satisfied as a pharmacist; and his attitude toward leaving pharmacy or changing to another type of work within the same profession. The pharmacist expresses his attitude toward his work. The referrant for such an attitude is his personal feeling, and whether the worker goes about his tasks Pagliacci-like with a mask of joy while reporting that he is dissatisfied with his work, or with a sullen countenance while reporting satisfaction, it is his feeling about his work that is important. A pharmacist may have a position, salary, and working conditions that others aspire to, but if he feels dissatisfied, it is his feeling with which we are concerned. While the conditions and circumstances are influential in shaping the attitude, and while the outward appearances of the individual usually reflect the inner feeling, it is the attitudes that serve as the frame of reference for the man's behavior, and these inner feelings are most directly accessible through the report of the subject.

Hoppock (25) used his Job Satisfaction Blank No. 1, from which the Pharmacy Satisfaction Scale has been adapted, in a study of teacher satisfaction. Working with 500 returns, he arranged the blanks in rank order of satisfaction (the method will be described below), and compared the 100 most satisfied with the 100 least satisfied. In this study, however, it was decided to establish a point on the continuum of satisfaction as the boundary between the two groups. All those whose responses placed them one-half negative deviation or more from the mean of satisfaction, in a normal distribution just under 31 per cent, were classified as dissatisfied. The remainder were included in the satisfied pharmacists group. For comparative purposes it is helpful to note that fewer than one third of the quantitative studies of satisfaction have yielded dissatisfied percentages in excess of 30 per cent. The median for the 133 percentages reported in all studies through the year 1947 as reported in a recent review (29) was 21 per cent.

What we thus obtain in this study are a group of "relatively satisfied" pharmacists and a group of "relatively dissatisfied" pharmacists. The former consists of some pharmacists who are satisfied "most of the time" rather than "all of the time," and who like it [pharmacy as an occupation] a good deal," but do not "love it." All but four of the satisfied indicate that they are glad they are pharmacists. Among the dissatisfied, however, more than half are glad they are pharmacists, but all of these in varying degrees show in their other responses less satisfaction than the "satisfied" group. It must be kept in mind in reading the remainder of this report that the dissatisfied group is, in fact, a group of relatively dissatisfied pharmacists, or of pharmacists relatively less satisfied than the satisfied pharmacists.

III Design of the Study

THIS chapter describes the materials used in the study, the method of selecting the subjects, and the mechanics of gathering the data. It concludes with a detailed statement on the size and characteristics of the sample of pharmacists.

MATERIALS USED IN GETTING DATA

To accomplish the objectives of the study it was necessary to have the pharmacists fill in the Strong Vocational Interest Blank as well as a scale that would indicate their feelings of satisfaction. Since the median time required by adult men to fill in the blank had been found to be thirty minutes (63:60) it was felt that a strong appeal would have to be made in a covering letter to overcome the resistance of the pharmacists to spending the necessary time on the two forms. Thus, each subject was sent one of the following:

1. A covering letter (Appendix) which emphasized the value of this study to pharmacy and sought to stimulate interest in returning the forms.

2. A stamped, self-addressed, return envelope.

3. The Strong Vocational Interest Blank for Men (Revised) Form M. As this instrument is well known and available in Strong (63), it is not described here.

4. The Pharmacy Satisfaction Scale (see Appendix). This is an adaptation of Hoppock's (25) Job Satisfaction Blank No. 1. The Pharmacy Satisfaction Scale contains several new sections: the upper third of the form, in which the pharmacist provides information on his occupational history and current status in the profession; the first subscale, in which the subject is to indicate if he is glad or sorry that he is a pharmacist; and the last section in which he is to comment if he desires an occupational change. A response item was added to Subscale E for those pharmacists who desired a change from one field to another within pharmacy. By the use of the Pharmacy Satisfaction Scale the members of the satisfied and dissatisfied groups were selected.

THE SUBJECTS

With the use of random numbers (14) the names of 1500 pharmacists were taken from the file of registered pharmacists of the New York State Board of Pharmacy in Albany. Pharmacists who were over sixty years of age, who had less than three years of experience, or who were residents of New York City, were excluded in so far as the records provided this information. The first two qualifications were applied to conform with the procedures used by Strong; the last was introduced to make the sampling as representative of the nation's pharmacists as possible.

The materials listed above were sent to each of the 1500 pharmacists. Within the next ten weeks three follow-up cards were sent to the same pharmacists at intervals of four, eight, and ten weeks after the mailing of the forms. Since most of the returns were anonymous in accordance with the instructions in the covering letter (it was felt that request for a name might discourage returns from small towns and villages and from dissatisfied employees in the cities), follow-ups had to be sent to all of the 1500. The use of a double follow-up postal card was very effective: many pharmacists returned the pre-addressed half of the card with a request for another set of forms, while others reported that the card had been a reminder and that they would fill out the forms at an early date. Some of the pharmacists wrote on these cards as others did on incomplete blanks that they returned, that they did not have the time to devote to them.

Arrangements were made for publicizing the study as a further stimulus to action by the subject pharmacists. A release appeared in many of the newspapers of the state within ten days after the materials were mailed. Feature articles appeared in Drug Topics and in the New York State Pharmacist, publication of the New York State Pharmaceutical Association, one and three months respectively after the mailing of the forms.

When it was apparent that the hoped-for goal of 500 usable returns would not be attained, it was decided to make an intensive personal solicitation for returns in one city, Utica, New York. This, it was felt, would serve several purposes. First, it would increase the total number of returns, an important factor in interest scale construction. Secondly, a high percentage sampling of one city would serve as a check on the adequacy of the statewide sampling, for if the Utica group contained a significantly higher percentage of dissatisfied, the state group

DESIGN OF THE STUDY 15

could not be expected to give an accurate representation of attitudes toward pharmacy. Finally, the interviews with the pharmacists, employers and employees, satisfied and dissatisfied, retail as well as hospital pharmacists, old and young, the prosperous and the not-so-prosperous, the chain store and the independent pharmacist, the downtown and the neighborhood druggist, would give meaning to the statistical data.

SIZE AND CHARACTERISTICS OF THE SAMPLE

Information on the size of the sample appears in Table 1. Of the 1500 forms mailed out, 464 or 31 per cent, were returned by mail. Thirty-seven more were secured through solicitation in Utica, making a total of 501 forms. Of this number, 450 were usable. Most of the remainder were too incomplete to be of value; a few came from men who had left the pharmaceutical occupations; and a few came from women whose given names were deceptively masculine (one from a pharmacist's wife who explained that she usually had to carry out these tasks for her husband or they were not done).

Twelve of the 464 forms returned by mail were from Utica. These 12 and the 37 from personal solicitation make a total of 49. This is a 61 per cent sample of the estimated 80 male pharmacists in Utica in 1947[1].

Table 1

SIZE OF SAMPLE

Forms mailed out	1500
Forms returned by mail	
Number	464
Per cent	31
Utica sample	
Forms received from Utica	12
Forms solicited in Utica	37
Total Utica sample	49
Percent of estimated total Utica population of pharmacists	61
Total forms received (mail or solicitation)	501
Total usable forms	450

---

1. Estimate made by the Utica Pharmacy Association.

The proportion of urban and rural pharmacists in the total sample (79.9 and 20.1 per cent) is so nearly identical with that in the total number of pharmacists in the United States as reported in the 16th Census, 1940 (80.3 and 19.7 per cent), that so far as community composition is concerned the sample is representative of the population of pharmacists.

No significant difference[2] was found in the percentages of dissatisfied in the 31 per cent sampling of New York State pharmacists and the 61 per cent sampling of Utica pharmacists. A further comparison of satisfaction in the two groups was made on the four subscales of the satisfaction scale used in determining the index of satisfaction. The critical ratios of the means of the Utica group and of a subsample of the statewide group were far short of significance. These data suggest that the 31 per cent sampling of New York State pharmacists represented by the mail returns provides as fair an estimate of degree of pharmacy satisfaction as we would have if the returns represented 61 per cent of these pharmacists.

To determine if any difference existed in the degree of satisfaction in the earlier and the later returns, a comparison was made of the responses of the first 262 returns with those of the next 177 on each of the four subscales. The differences did not even approach significance; the probability that these two groups belong to the same population for the largest observed difference in means (the second subscale) exceeded 35 per cent.

Although these tests indicate that there is consistency in the degree of satisfaction between the earlier and later returns in the total group, and between the total and the Utica group returns, there is the possibility that the sample of pharmacists, and particularly of satisfied pharmacists, is a biased one. The sample consists only of those pharmacists who voluntarily returned the forms. Among the pharmacists who failed to participate (even among the relatively small group of Utica pharmacists, 39 per cent of the total, who failed to submit their forms), there could be a far higher percentage of dissatisfied than in the total sample.

---

2. Significance in the difference of means is determined by the formula $D/\sigma_d = \frac{M_1 - M_2}{\sqrt{\sigma_{M_1}^2 + \sigma_{M_2}^2}}$. D/σ_d must equal or exceed 1.96 for significance at the .05 level. All tests of significance in this study will be at the .05 level.

IV Differentiating Characteristics of the Satisfied and Dissatisfied

THIS chapter describes the technique of measuring the professed satisfaction of pharmacists. It reports on the differences between the total group of satisfied and dissatisfied pharmacists, and between the 50 most and 50 least satisfied pharmacists. Finally, it summarizes and evaluates the reasons given for dissatisfaction.

THE TECHNIQUE OF MEASURING PHARMACY SATISFACTION

Following the procedure used by Hoppock (25) the mean and standard deviation were computed for each of the four subscales (B,C,D, and E) of the Pharmacy Satisfaction Scale. A numerical value was assigned to each of the possible responses on the subscales. In subscale B, for example, eleven numbers were assigned, starting with one for the "I hate it" response and ending with 11 for the "I love it" response. The mean and the standard deviation were then computed for each subscale. Then the deviation from the mean of each man's response on each of the four subscales was divided by sigma to secure a scale value. The deviations in the direction of satisfaction were given a positive value; those in the opposite direction, negative. The scale values for each of the four subscales were then summed to secure an index of satisfaction for each pharmacist.

The satisfaction indices of the pharmacists were then placed in order from the highest positive to the highest negative index. The mean and sigma were computed. All pharmacists whose index was at least one-half negative deviation from the mean were classified as "dissatisfied"; those above that point, as "satisfied." The former group included 117, or 26 per cent of the 450 usable pharmacy blanks.

Of the 450 pharmacists only 50, or 11 per cent, said that they were sorry they were pharmacists. Forty-six of these were among the 117 dissatisfied pharmacists. Four of the satisfied pharmacists were sorry they were pharmacists. One of these four was sorry because it was not "financially worth what you are putting into it; i.e., just look at the remunerations from dentistry, medicine, or law." Another one complained about some of the "unethical" practices. It is important to note that while these same complaints were made by many of the dissatisfied pharmacists whether "sorry" or not, and by some of the satisfied pharmacists who were not sorry, the satisfied pharmacists tended to like their work more, for longer periods of time, etc., than the dissatisfied. Being sorry that one is in a certain occupation does not necessarily make for dissatisfaction with one's work; likewise, being glad that one is in a certain occupation does not necessarily make for satisfaction with one's work. We are concerned here with attitudes towards one's work, and it is these that are used in classification according to satisfaction.

NONDIFFERENTIATING CHARACTERISTICS

Various facts about the background, experience, and occupation of the pharmacists were made available through the information on the upper portion of the satisfaction scale. This was the only source of such data, for the similar but less pertinent questions on the first page of the Vocational Interest Blank were hidden by the Satisfaction Scale which had been stapled upon it. The 333 satisfied and 117 dissatisfied pharmacists were compared as to these characteristics to determine if these two groups whose likes and dislikes were to be contrasted were different in background. Critical ratios of the means or of percentages were computed, and no significant differences were found for the following (Table 2): average age; World War II veteran status, number having relatives in pharmacy, occupation in pharmacy (i.e., owner, member of corporation, employee), percentage urban and rural; and average years of experience. The percentages of retail employees working for chain stores, in the two groups, were nearly identical: 16.30 and 16.37 per cent.

Age

Hoppock (26) found that there was a slight tendency for job satisfaction to rise as workers advanced in age. This is not surprising, for in a different study (25) the same author reported that a worker's job satisfaction increases as he rises on the occupational ladder. Two more recent surveys reveal an increase: one after the age of 26 (72); the other, after 29 (2); Super (66) likewise reported an increase in satisfaction with age, but cyclical in nature, with the age groups of 24 - 34 and 45 - 54 feeling less satisfied than others. This too was in

DIFFERENTIATING CHARACTERISTICS

general agreement with his finding that the percentage of satisfied men increases with occupational level. It seemed advisable, therefore, to compare not merely the average age of the two groups, but also the percentages of the satisfied and

Table 2

NONDIFFERENTIATING CHARACTERISTICS OF 333 SATISFIED AND 117 DISSATISFIED PHARMACISTS

Characteristic	Dissatisfied Mean	%	Satisfied Mean	%	Difference	D/σ_d [a]
Age	40.31		41.24		0.93	0.94
World War II veteran status		25.89		20.74	5.15	1.10
Relative in pharmacy		33.91		27.44	6.47	1.29
Urban employment		81.81		79.23	2.58	0.59
Years in pharmacy	20.32		21.08		0.76	0.72
Occupation in pharmacy						
Owner		45.69		49.85	4.16	0.77
Member of corporation		4.31		7.90	3.59	1.49
Employee		50.00		42.25	7.75	1.44

a. In this and subsequent tables, D/σ_d is the ratio of the difference in means of two groups, and of the standard error of the difference. For example, the D/σ_d for the characteristic of age can be simply stated as:

$$\frac{\text{mean age of satisfied - mean age of dissatisfied}}{\text{standard error of the difference}}$$

In this study, D/σ_d, or the critical ratio, as it is frequently called, must equal or exceed 1.96 to be regarded as significant; that is, a difference in the means of the two samples (e.g., satisfied and dissatisfied) must be sufficiently large that such difference could be expected by chance alone in only 5 or less times in every 100 comparisons of samples drawn from the same population.

the dissatisfied for each age group: 20 - 29; 30 - 39; 40 - 49; 50 - 59 (Table 3). The differences were not significant. Still another age breakdown was made: 20 - 23; 24 - 34; 35 - 44; 45 - 54; 55 plus. Unlike Super's findings, the satisfied had a higher percentage than the dissatisfied in the age groups 24 - 34 and 45 - 54, as they did in all the groupings except 35 - 44. None of these differences, however, was significant.

Table 3

DIFFERENCES IN PERCENTAGES OF SATISFIED AND DISSATISFIED PHARMACISTS FOR VARIOUS AGE GROUPS

Age Group	Dissatisfied Number	%	Satisfied Number	%	Difference	D/σd
20 - 29	15	12.83	31	9.45	3.38	0.97
30 - 39	37	31.63	115	35.06	3.41	0.68
40 - 49	49	41.88	116	35.37	6.51	1.24
50 - 59	14	11.96	62	18.90	6.94	1.88
60 -	2	1.70	4	1.22	0.48	0.03
Total	117	100.00	328[a]	100.00		
20 - 23			4	1.22	1.22	0.11
24 - 34	27	23.10	74	22.55	0.55	0.12
35 - 44	58	49.57	143	43.60	5.97	1.11
45 - 54	24	20.50	81	24.70	4.20	0.95
55 -	8	6.83	26	7.93	1.10	0.38
Total	117	100.00	328[a]	100.00		

a. Five satisfied pharmacists (total number, 333) failed to give their age.

TWO DIFFERENTIATING AREAS

Significant differences were found between the two total groups (satisfied and dissatisfied) in two major areas: the nature of the organization in which the pharmacist was working (regardless whether as employer, member of corporation, or employee); and the percentage of his time devoted to prescription or research as contrasted with sales or management (Table 4). A higher percentage of the dissatisfied, approximately 96 per cent, were engaged in retail pharmacy, as compared with 88 per cent of the satisfied. The difference is significant. A higher percentage of the satisfied than the dissatisfied were in pharmacy manufacturing and in hospitals, with the differences significant in the former and very nearly so in the latter. Reltively few pharmacists were involved in these last two comparisons, only 21 in manufacturing and 20 in hospital work.

Table 4

DIFFERENTIATING CHARACTERISTICS OF 333 SATISFIED AND 117 DISSATISFIED PHARMACISTS

Characteristics	Dissatisfied Mean	%	Satisfied Mean	%	Difference	D/σd
Nature of organization						
Retail		95.65		87.73	7.92	3.01
Manufacturing		1.75		5.84	4.09	2.29
Hospital		1.75		5.53	3.78	1.92
Wholesale		0.85		0.90	0.05	0.05
Percentage of time on prescription	28.80		36.80		8.00	3.04
0 - 25		64.34		46.91	17.43	3.33
26 - 75		27.83		41.36	13.53	2.71
76 - 100		7.83		11.73	3.90	1.27

When the mean percentage of prescription work is computed for the two groups, about 29 per cent for the dissatisfied and 37 per cent for the satisfied, the difference is significant. Likewise, the differences are significant when the frequencies of the two groups for 0 - 25 and 26 - 75 per cent prescription work are compared, with a higher percentage of the dissatisfied in the first category and of the satisfied in the second. No significant difference was found in the 76 - 100 per cent prescription groups.

It was originally planned that pharmacists devoting only 0 - 25 per cent of their time to prescription or research would be classified as business pharmacists, and those spending 76 - 100 per cent as apothecary pharmacists. Because the latter group was too small, it was redefined to consist of all those devoting 26 - 100 per cent of their time to prescription work, making the two groups nearly equal in size (Apothecary, 188; Business, 194; 42 of the returns were not classifiable as apothecary or business, the percentage of prescription work being unindicated or the response ambiguous; and 26 of those classifiable could not be used because the Interest Blanks were inadequately filled in for weighting purposes). A comparison of the satisfaction of the two groups, with about 81 per cent of the apothecaries and only 70 per cent of the business pharmacists satisfied, yields a significant critical ratio (Table 5).

Table 5

SATISFACTION IN APOTHECARY AND BUSINESS PHARMACIST GROUPS[a]

Number	Apothecary	Business	Difference	$D/\sigma d$
Total	188	194		
Satisfied	152	135		
Percentage satisfied	80.85	69.58	11.27	2.58

a. Of the 450 usable returns, 42 could not be classified as apothecary or business, and 26 were inadequately filled in for use in weighting.

DIFFERENTIATING CHARACTERISTICS

Of the 17 characteristics of the pharmacists on which data were obtained in this study, only five in the following two areas yield significant differences between the satisfied and the dissatisfied: the nature of the organization in which engaged and the percentage of prescription work. A significantly higher percentage of the dissatisfied tend to be in retail pharmacy, and, within retail work, to be engaged for a greater part of the time in business or sales tasks than are the satisfied. On the other hand, there is no significant difference in the type of position in which the satisfied and the dissatisfied are engaged, whether owner, member of corporation, or employee.

These findings must be considered in the light of several other facts. Forty-seven of the satisfied pharmacists devote only 0 - 25 per cent of their time to prescription work. About 36 per cent of the dissatisfied are in the 26 - 75 or 76 - 100 per cent prescription groups. In differentiating the apothecary and business groups, all those pharmacists who had already been classified as dissatisfied and who had indicated on the satisfaction scale that their dissatisfaction was the result of too little or too much prescription work, were excluded from the apothecary-business classifications; that is, a dissatisfied pharmacist in the 0 - 25 per cent category who claimed he was dissatisfied due to the inadequate amount of prescription work in his job was not classified as prescription or business. Relatively few such cases were found: few dissatisfied pharmacists blamed their unfavorable attitudes on the limited prescription function of their job. Of the 42 pharmacists unclassified as to percentage of prescription, 25 were satisfied. Of these, 9 preferred more and 8 preferred less prescription work. Of the 17 dissatisfied pharmacists, 11 preferred more and 4 preferred less prescription. Of the total 117 dissatisfied pharmacists only 11 suggested that their dissatisfaction was because of too little prescription work. It therefore seems doubtful that frustration of ambition for prescription work is a widespread factor in dissatisfaction among pharmacists.

DIFFERENTIATING CHARACTERISTICS OF
THE 50 MOST AND 50 LEAST SATISFIED

When the two groups at the extremes of satisfaction are compared the results are somewhat different. Among the 50 most satisfied pharmacists 100 per cent respond that they are glad they are pharmacists. Among the 50 most dissatisfied, 20 per cent are glad, 8 per cent make no response, and 72 per cent are sorry. The latter figure is to be contrasted with the 38 per cent of the total dissatisfied group that reports it is sorry.

As in the comparison between the two total groups, no significance was found in the difference between the percentages having relatives in pharmacy, or living in urban or rural areas.

In both comparisons the percentage of World War II veterans was higher in the dissatisfied group, though in neither case was the difference significant. The percentages in the first case were 26 per cent and 21 per cent for the dissatisfied and the satisfied respectively, and in the subgroup comparison, 31 and 16 per cent. It was to be expected, in the comparisons of subgroups in which the average age of the dissatisfied was significantly lower than among the satisfied, that the percentage of veterans, a function of age, would also be higher.

Age and Experience

A sharp difference appears in the age composition of the two extreme groups (Table 6). The mean age of the satisfied is about 45; that of the dissatisfied, 40.

Table 6

AGE DISTRIBUTION OF 50 LEAST AND 50 MOST SATISFIED PHARMACISTS

Age	Least Satisfied Number	%	Most Satisfied Number	%
20 - 29	7	14	3	6
30 - 39	16	32	9	18
40 - 49	21	42	21	42
50 - 59	6	12	16	32
60 -			1	2
Total	50	100	50	100
Mean	39.90		45.10	
Difference		5.20		
$D/\sigma d$		2.88		

DIFFERENTIATING CHARACTERISTICS

Likewise, the dissatisfied group averaged only about 20 years of experience in contrast with the mean of 27 years of experience of the satisfied group (Table 7). In the comparison of the total groups, these two characteristics, age and length of experience, showed differences that were clearly insignificant, whereas in the comparison of the two extreme subgroups the differences are significant.

Table 7

YEARS IN PHARMACY OF 50 LEAST AND 50 MOST SATISFIED PHARMACISTS

Years	Least Satisfied	Most Satisfied
1 - 2	2	1
3 - 4		
5 - 9	5	1
10 - 14	8	5
15 - 19	6	7
20 - 29	24	14
30 - 39	5	17
40 -		5
Total	50	50
Mean	19.93	26.79
Difference		6.86
$D/\sigma d$		3.61

Prescription Work

The mean percentage of prescription work is substantially higher for the satisfied in both comparisons, but it is even higher for the satisfied and lower for the dissatisfied in the comparison of the two extreme subgroups than in the other comparisons (Table 8). The difference between the average percentage of prescription work of the two is greater, and the critical ratio larger. The critical ratios of the percentages of those engaged in prescription work 0 - 25 per cent and 76 - 100 per cent of the time are both significant and larger than the comparable ratios between the two larger groups.

A shift occurs when the data of the subgroups are analyzed. Unlike the more heterogeneous satisfaction groups, between the extreme groups there is no significant difference in the number of pharmacists devoting 26 - 75 per cent of their time in prescription work, while there is a difference in the 76 - 100 per cent groups. Thus, when the two extreme groups are compared, the relationship between percentage of prescription and satisfaction becomes more clear-cut. The percentages of satisfied pharmacists who spend more than 25 per cent of their time in

Table 8

PERCENTAGE OF TIME SPENT ON PRESCRIPTION WORK OF SATISFIED AND DISSATISFIED PHARMACISTS IN STANDARDIZATION GROUP AND EXTREME SUBGROUPS

Per Cent of Time Spent on Prescription Work	Dissatisfied	Satisfied	Difference	$D/\sigma d$
0 - 25%				
Standardization	64.4	46.9	17.5	3.33
Subgroups	71.4	37.5	33.9	3.55
26 - 75%				
Standardization	27.8	41.4	13.6	2.71
Subgroups	26.5	43.8	17.3	1.81
76 - 100%				
Standardization	7.8	11.7	3.9	1.27
Subgroups	2.1	18.7	16.6	2.78

DIFFERENTIATING CHARACTERISTICS

prescription work are 53 for the total satisfied group and 63 for the extreme subgroup. Comparable figures for the dissatisfied are 36 and 29 per cent. The difference between the satisfied and the dissatisfied in the number spending more than 25 per cent of the time in prescription work is 17 per cent for the total groups and 34 per cent for the extreme subgroups.

Occupation in Pharmacy

Analysis of the data on the occupation in pharmacy shows the same clarification as we move to the more homogeneous groups (Table 9). In the total group of dissatisfied there are a smaller percentage of owners and a larger percentage of employees than in the satisfied group. In neither case is the difference significant. In the subgroups, however, the differences are greater, and the critical ratio of the percentage of owners is significant.

The differences between the satisfied and the dissatisfied in the percentage in retail and manufacturing that were reliable in the criterion group are maintained in the comparison of the two subgroups. Because of the smaller size of the subgroups, however, the differences are not significant.

In summary, then, the characteristics in which the subgroups of the 50 most satisfied and the 50 least satisfied differ significantly are (1) age, the satisfied being older; (2) experience in pharmacy, the satisfied having longer experience; (3) percentage of prescription work involved in their current occupation, the satisfied having a higher percentage; (4) the occupation of owner in pharmacy, a higher percentage of the satisfied being

Table 9

OCCUPATION IN PHARMACY OF 50 LEAST AND 50 MOST SATISFIED PHARMACISTS

Occupation	Least Satisfied Number	%	Most Satisfied Number	%	Difference	D/σd
Owner	25	50	30	72	22	2.32
Member of corporation	3	6	3	6		
Employee	22	44	11	22	22	1.20

so engaged. The fact that the extreme dissatisfaction group can be differentiated from the extreme satisfaction group by three characteristics (age, experience, and occupation in pharmacy) that do not differentiate the total groups suggests the possibility that the total groups may be too heterogeneous. This may bear heavily upon our success in differentiating their vocational interests.

REASONS FOR DISSATISFACTION

Subscale F of the Pharmacy Satisfaction Scale seeks evidence of the specific type of change desired by those pharmacists, satisfied or not, who wish to shift their "line of work within pharmacy or a change from pharmacy to another field." Few of the satisfied made any response. Many, but not all, of the dissatisfied used these few lines either to indicate a change or, more frequently, to complain about certain conditions in pharmacy. These remarks are valuable because they are spontaneous and, in large measure, unstructured. They contribute to a clinical picture of the dissatisfied pharmacist. If they are classified for statistical treatment they form more categories than it is possible to deal with meaningfully. It is more fruitful to note the trends in their responses, for this throws light not only upon the attitudes of dissatisfied pharmacists, but also upon our concepts of satisfaction.

Two criticisms of pharmacy appear most frequently. These it should be noted, are made not merely by the dissatisfied but also by some of the satisfied pharmacists. Foremost is the objection to the long hours of work of the retail pharmacist, in which connection it is suggested that the working day be reduced and that Sunday and holiday hours be eliminated. About one third of all the dissatisfied specifically complain about this condition, and, as suggested more fully below, it may be that the request for a change in many other cases simply masks dissatisfaction with the work week. Typical comments follow:

1. A 34-year-old owner of a non-chain pharmacy, in a rural resort area, with 12 years experience, 0 - 25 per cent prescription: "A business where I could have regular hours and a holiday would mean that I would be free as most other people are. Preferably either in manufacturing or as a wholesaler."

2. A 55-year-old employee in pharmacy manufacturing in a large city, 34 years experience, 26 - 75 per cent prescription: "My own boss in a small ethical retail and physicians manufacturing pharmacy. The greatest detriment to pharmacy is the long hours in the business."

DIFFERENTIATING CHARACTERISTICS

3. A 28-year-old owner of a non-chain retail store, 7 years experience, 0 - 25 per cent prescription: "Research or manufacturing. Any profession yielding public respect and satisfactory return for the investment in time and money."

4. A 42-year-old employee in a non-chain retail pharmacy in a small city, 21 years experience, 26 - 75 per cent prescription: "Medical field representative for [large pharmaceutical manufacturing firms mentioned] where you have Saturdays, Sundays and holidays free and your vacation without bickering."

The desire to change to wholesale or manufacturing pharmacy is so frequently expressed by those who complain about the length of the work week that it is impossible to know if the expressed desire to change to manufacturing, wholesale, research, or even non-pharmacy occupations unaccompanied by explanation as to the motive does not really reflect dissatisfaction with this condition of pharmacy. It may well be that this condition, long characteristic of the profession, has taken on a semblance of immutability, despite wartime reduction in hours, and has led many of the dissatisfied to a "devil's horn" effect whereby rejection of this undesirable characteristic of pharmacy has led to the rejection of pharmacy itself or of the current occupation in pharmacy.

A second theme that runs through the complaints expresses the desire to work for an "ethical" or "professional" organization. This appears in more than 10 per cent of the Satisfaction Scales of the dissatisfied.

A change to pharmaceutical manufacturing is desired more than any other intrapharmacy change. Approximately 13 per cent express a preference for such work. If these pharmacists, and the smaller number who request a change to wholesale or sales work want these changes as an escape from long hours, then the dissatisfaction that exists in our total group can be attributed in the majority of the cases to the length of the work week.

In contrast to complaints about hours, relatively few criticized their earnings. Again, many who desired occupational changes within or outside pharmacy may have been seeking higher salaries, but such an inference seems less justified in the case of income than of hours because of the fewer explicit references to salary. Other investigations of the correlates of job satisfaction have yielded conflicting results. Seidman and Watson (47) report that of 157 men who rated their most interesting job, 132 gave salary as the least important of eight factors. Vocational aspiration, congenial work conditions and social contacts, and initiative, responsibility, and prestige headed the list of factors. More recently, Habbe (21), studying the attitudes of life insurance salesmen, found no significant relationship between earnings and job satisfaction. Two other recent reports (2, 34), however, give evidence of a significant relationship. One of these, by Kerr (34), on two studies involving 13,000 industrial workers, supports the view that earnings are a highly important factor in labor turnover. These contradictory findings can be explained only in terms of such variables as the nature of the study, the form and content of the questionnaire, occupational level of the subjects, the extent of trade union organization, management-employee relationships, current cost of living, and the existence of one or more extremely unattractive characteristics (e.g., long hours) that might overshadow other grievances.

Approximately 10 per cent desired changes in the direction of more "scientific" work, such as "research," chemistry, medicine (only two), hospital work. While it is impossible to know the thinking of those who prefer to work in a "professional" or "ethical" pharmacy, it is likely that many of them desired more prescription work.

A higher percentage of the dissatisfied desired changes in the direction of sales and management work rather than toward prescription. Even excluding the interest in pharmaceutical manufacturing (the underlying motive is uncertain, as it could be shorter hours, pay, research, or sales), the percentage preferring the business fields is at least 15. This includes wholesale business, "management duties," and self-ownership, as well as business occupations outside pharmacy, such as real estate, clerical work, operating a small hotel, and the sale of large items such as furniture.

If we are to make inferences as to the origin of dissatisfaction from among the remarks concerning pharmacy made in subscale F, we must say that it is caused either by (1) working conditions or (2) misplacement within the profession. The criticisms of working conditions in pharmacy suggest that the pharmacists want the advantages of a business (short hours) with those of a profession (pay and especially prestige). They report that they have long hours, low prestige, and, in fewer cases, low pay.

There is little evidence of a deeper maladjustment among the scales containing criticisms of pharmacy. Only one person complained about a dictatorial superior, a complaint which might have been well founded. The five who desire ownership

DIFFERENTIATING CHARACTERISTICS 31

of a store could be seeking escape from a subordinate function. It is only when we examine the scales in which the pharmacists express desires for change outside the profession that there is more foundation for questioning the general adjustment of the individual, and then only in a small minority of the cases. The data in this study do not support the view of Fisher and Hanna (15) that "a large part of vocational maladjustment. . . . is but a reflection of emotional maladjustment."

Without further information about the individual one cannot treat the desire to transfer to the real estate business or horticulture as anything but an occupational preference. A 31-year-old pharmacy employee whose father is a pharmacist writes: "I wanted to be a journalist or a writer, but was born into pharmacy." This case, like several others, suggests vocational misplacement. But there is reason to suspect the following responses as escapes from reality, including the routine nature of many tasks:

> Travel, at a decent salary
> Spending a rich man's money
> Anything in music or sporting goods
> Clerical work
> Aviation--if I were younger
> Creating something
> Writing

Analysis of the reasons for dissatisfaction suggests that it is generated by (1) conditions in pharmacy, especially the long work week; (2) misplacement within pharmacy which in some cases may be a reaction to these working conditions; (3) misplacement in pharmacy with preference for a non-pharmacy occupation, which also in some cases may be a reaction to working conditions in pharmacy; (4) maladjustment of the individual which is reflected in unrealistic or immature preferences.

V Construction of Three Pharmacy Interest Scales

THE methods used in establishing the scales were, with certain important exceptions described below, the same as those used by Strong (63: 74 - 76). The "like" (L), "indifferent" (I), and "dislike" (D) responses on each of the 400 items of the Vocational Interest Blank were tallied for 450 pharmacists and then expressed in the form of percentages. Separate tallies were recorded for each of the six groups: Apothecary-Satisfied; Business-Satisfied; Unclassified-Satisfied; Apothecary-Dissatisfied; Business-Dissatisfied; Unclassified-Dissatisfied. At the completion of this task there were 18 different percentages for each of the 400 items, that is, L, I, and D percentage for each of the six groups.

ESTABLISHING WEIGHTS FOR EACH ITEM

The percentages were sent to Strong's Vocational Interest Research Project where weights were calculated for each item for each of the three scales by computing the difference between these percentages and those of the group used as point of reference. In establishing the Vocational Interest Scale for Pharmacists, for example, the percentage of satisfied pharmacists who made an L response to any item were compared with the percentage of the men-in-general group that had expressed such liking. By entering a table (designed by Strong to expedite the procedure of weighting) with these two percentages it was possible to read off the weight given the L response to this one item on this scale. The greater the difference between the percentages (pharmacists and men-in-general), the greater the weight accorded that particular item. The weights range from -4 to +4 the sign depending on whether the percentage of liking, disliking, or indifferent of the group in question (pharmacists) exceeds or is less than that for the base (men-in-general) group. Thus, if the percentage of satisfied pharmacists who circled the L response on any one item exceeded that of the men-in-general group sufficiently to be assigned the weight, the weight would be a positive one; and if the satisfied pharmacists' percentage were smaller, the weight would be negative. The same procedure was used in weighting the I and D responses to this item, and in weighting the three possible responses to each of the remaining items on the blank.

CONSTRUCTION OF THREE PHARMACY SCALES

While the procedure was exactly the same in determining weights for the Satisfied vs. Dissatisfied Pharmacists Scale and the Apothecary vs. Business Pharmacists Scale, the groups that were contrasted were different. In the case of the former scale, the percentage of satisfied pharmacists who made an L response to any item was compared with the percentage of dissatisfied pharmacists who had expressed such liking. Then by use of the same table the weight was found for this response on this item. The same method was followed in weighting the I and D responses for this item, and all three possible responses to all the remaining items in the blank.

In the case of the Apothecary vs. Business Pharmacists Scale the percentage of apothecary pharmacists who made an L response to an item was contrasted with that of the business pharmacists. Again the table was used to assign the weight to the item. The weight was negative if the percentage of apothecary pharmacists who liked it was less than that of business pharmacists, and positive if apothecary liking exceeded business pharmacists liking. The weights were similarly determined for the responses to each of the 400 items in the blank.

Taking one item as an illustration of the weights in our three scales, a substantially higher percentage of pharmacists than men-in-general like the occupation "Buyer of Merchandise." The L response was therefore assigned a weight of +4. A smaller but still substantial percentage of men-in-general than pharmacists were indifferent to or disliked it: the I and D responses were weighted minus two. On the Satisfied vs. Dissatisfied Pharmacists Scale, the L, I, and D responses to this same item were weighted 1, -1, and O respectively, because a slightly higher percentage of the satisfied than of the dissatisfied liked it and a slightly smaller percentage was indifferent to it. There was no significant difference in the D percentages of the two. On the Apothecary vs. Business Pharmacists Scale all the responses to this item have zero weights, for there was no significant difference in the percentages of the two groups.

STABILITY OF A WEIGHT

The stability of an interest weight, important to both the reliability and validity of the scale, depends upon the consistency of an individual's response to an item. The weight of plus four assigned to the L response to the item "Buyer of Merchandise" on the Pharmacy Scale is stable to the extent that in retaking the Vocational Interest Blank our satisfied pharmacists (criterion group) score as high a percentage of liking as before; and that the men-in-general group scores as low a percentage as before. This of course depends upon constancy of response of the members of the group.

In his discussion of the stability of interest items Strong (63:666) reports on a study of the shifts in response to an item between test and retest on the Interest Blank. When an individual changes his response from $\underline{L}$ to $\underline{I}$ or $\underline{I}$ to $\underline{D}$ or vice versa, he is credited with a single shift; when he changes from $\underline{L}$ to $\underline{D}$ or vice versa, it is a double shift. The maximum number of shifts possible on any item is two, the minimum is zero, and the number which will occur by chance is .89. The average number of shifts for each of 25 college students who filled in the blank a second time after a one-year interval was only .37 per item. Strong also refers to a study by Burnham[1] in which coefficients of stability were computed for the items of the blank. His subjects were college students retested after intervals of one week and three years. For every item the coefficient of stability exceeded chance. The mean coefficient of stability for all the items was 72 over one week and 62 over three years compared with the coefficient of 43 for chance.

These studies suggest that item responses have considerable stability. Since the subjects in both studies were students, many of them still experiencing the developmental changes of late adolescence with their effects upon interest, it seems justifiable to regard reported item constancy as a minimum estimate for scales used with adults.

VARIATIONS FROM USUAL CONSTRUCTION PROCEDURES

Table 10 indicates which groups were used for weight and standardization purposes, and as points of reference. The variations from the usual procedure in constructing a vocational scale for the Vocational Interest Blank are as follows:

1. The Vocational Interest Scale for Pharmacists, most nearly like the standard scales in its construction, differs from the occupational scales developed by Strong in that all the dissatisfied have been excluded from the weight and norm groups. Strong's procedure has been to discard blanks from those who voluntarily indicated dissatisfaction, for example by their

---

1. P. S. Burnham, "Stability of Interest Test Scores" (unpublished doctoral dissertation, Yale University, 1935).

CONSTRUCTION OF THREE PHARMACY SCALES

statement that they were considering some other type of work[2]. But this is very different from the systematic attempt in this study to seek out such information. The Vocational Interest Scale for Pharmacists will henceforth be referred to as the Pharmacy Scale.

2. The Satisfied vs. Dissatisfied Pharmacists Scale (abbreviated hereafter to the S-D Scale) also used only the satisfied pharmacists for weight and norm purposes; in addition, it substituted the dissatisfied for men-in-general as the point of reference.

3. The Apothecary vs. Business Pharmacists Scale (abbreviated to the A-B Scale) used only the apothecary pharmacists, those devoting more than 25 per cent of their time to prescription work, for weight and norm purposes; in addition, it substituted the business pharmacists, those devoting 0 - 25 per cent of their time to prescription work, for men-in-general as the point of reference.

SIZE OF WEIGHT AND NORM GROUPS

Except for the variables that were being investigated, explained below, the techniques used here conform with those used by Strong. The same procedures were followed in weighting and in standardizing the scales. In the three scales (see Table 10) the same group was used in standardizing the scale as in determining the weights. This procedure was introduced, at the cost of having to get additional returns to validate the study, because there has been abundant evidence that increase in the size of the criterion group at least to 250, preferably to 300, and if possible to 500, considerably decreases sampling errors (3, 18, 63). Strong wrote: "If one has available date on 200 or on 500 cases, is it better to build a scale on half of these and develop the norms from the other half, or to use all the cases for constructing the scale and base the norms also on the same cases? All the data suggest that the larger the criterion group upon which the scale is based the better. The second procedure is therefore preferable." (63:650).

Both of the contrasted groups, the criterion and the point of reference group, should meet this quantitative standard if the results are to be staisfactory. The Pharmacy Scale is built upon a criterion group of 313 and a men-in-general group of

---

2. Personal communication from Dr. E. K. Strong, Jr., May 10, 1947.

nearly 5000 cases, "beyond suspicion as far as size is concerned" (63:649). The sampling error in this scale should be far less than that for the S-D Scale in which the comparable numbers are 313 and 111, and the A-B Scale, 188 and 194.

ESTABLISHING NORMS

After the weights had been established for each possible response to each item on the blank, for each of the three scales (Pharmacy Scale, S-D Scale, A-B Scale), the blanks of all the members of the norm group were scored. Then the mean and standard deviation of the raw scores were computed for each of the three scales.

Table 10

COMPOSITION OF THE THREE NEW PHARMACY SCALES

Scale	Weight Group	Norm Group	Point of Reference
Vocational Interest Scale for Pharmacists	All satisfied pharmacists: N-313[a]	All satisfied pharmacists: N-313	Men-in-general Strong's P-1
Satisfied vs. Dissatisfied Pharmacists Scale	All satisfied pharmacists: N-313	All satisfied pharmacists: N-313	All dissatisfied pharmacists: N-111
Apothecary vs. Business Pharmacists Scale	All apothecary pharmacists: N-188	All apothecary pharmicists: N-188	All business pharmicsts: N-194

a. The groups of 333 satisfied and of 117 dissatisfied pharmacists used in the study of background variables were reduced to 313 and 111 members respectively when some of the Strong Vocational Interest Blanks were found to be inadequately filled in.

CONSTRUCTION OF THREE PHARMACY SCALES

In accordance with the usual procedure they were converted into standard scores, and these in turn were given letter grade equivalents. The norms for each of the three scales are given in Table 11.

Table 11

SCORES AND LETTER GRADES FOR THREE PHARMACY SCALES

	Pharmacists Scale	Raw Scores S-D Scale	A-B Scale	Standard Scores	Letter Grades
	145			76	A
	135	100		73	A
	133	98	70	72	A
	125	93	65	70	A
	110	78	53	65	A
	95	65	43	60	A
	78	50	30	55	A
Mean	60	35	18	50	A
	45	21	5	45	A
	28	8	-5	40	B+
	13	-8	-18	35	B
	-5	-20	-30	30	B-
	-20	-35	-43	25	C+
	-33	-50	-53	20	C
	-43	-55	-58	18	C
		-72	-72	12	C
			-77	10	C
Sigma	32.43	28.42	23.71		

CONSTRUCTION OF THREE PHARMACY SCALES

The mean raw score of each group was arbitrarily assigned a standard score of 50, and sigma was given the value of 10 standard score points. Then the letter grade of A was assigned to all scores one-half negative deviation from the mean and above, or all standard scores of 45 and above. The other standard score equivalents of letter grades are shown in Table 12, together with the percentages of the criterion group within each grade category. The letter grades as well as the standard scores on the three scales have the same statistical meaning as Strong's.

The higher mean raw score of the norm group on the Pharmacy Scale, as compared with the other two, points to the greater contrast in interests between pharmacists and men-in-general than between satisfied and dissatisfied pharmacists or apothecary and business pharmacists. The correspondingly larger sigma shows the greater variability in this contrast, and is also a function of the greater variation that comes from increasing the size of the groups. In keeping with this, we find that the Pharmacy Scale gives a higher percentage of A and C scores than the other two.

Table 12

PERCENTAGE OF NORM GROUP IN EACH SCORING CATEGORY ON THREE PHARMACY SCALES

Letter Grade	Standard Score	Pharmacists Scale	Percentages S-D Scale	A-B Scale
A	45 and above	72.20	66.45	67.55
B+	40 to 44	11.82	16.93	17.02
B	35 39	9.58	10.22	9.58
B-	30 34	3.20	3.84	2.66
C+	25 29	1.92	2.24	3.19
C	24 and below	1.28	0.32	

VI Effectiveness of the Scales

THE methods used to test the validity of the hypotheses are described in this chapter and the results reported. The reliability of the scores and stability of the items are discussed.

THE VALIDATION SAMPLE

The 105 sets of forms used to test the hypotheses of the study were filled in by 60 pharmacists from Connecticut, 42 from New York, two from Massachusetts, and one from New Hampshire. The Connecticut forms were obtained at a meeting of the New Haven Druggists' Association; the others were requested and received through the mail[1] as in the case of the original New York State group.

The validation and standardization groups differ in that the latter contains only New York State pharmacists. Since cultural factors and pharmacist certification requirements in Connecticut are similar to those in New York, the different geographical makeup of the two groups is probably not important. The gap of eighteen months between the time the original and the validation groups filled in the forms may have some bearing on the satisfaction of the members, especially since living costs had risen. One Connecticut pharmacist, for example, who indicated he was satisfied a good deal of the time, added the phrase "until recent conditions." Although the New Haven pharmacists, members of a professional organization, constituted a select group, there was no significance in the difference between the percentage of dissatisfied in that group and in the randomly selected New York State standardization group.

The total validation group of 105 pharmacists was subdivided into satisfied and dissatisfied groups with 71 and 32 members respectively (two of the returns could not be classified) and into apothecary and business pharmacists groups with 49 and 48 members (eight returns were unclassifiable). The percentage of dissatisfied pharmacists in the validation group was not significantly different from that in the original group. Differences

---

[1]. Of the 150 sets of forms sent to New York State pharmacists in establishing the validation group, 45 were returned, 43 of them usable. Of the forms sent by the Massachusetts College of Pharmacy to 50 alumni, only three were returned.

between the satisfied and dissatisfied groups of validation pharmacists were significant for the following background characteristics: percentage of prescription work (with the satisfied so engaged about 42 per cent of the time, and the dissatisfied, 25 per cent); the percentage of pharmacists engaged in prescription work 0 - 25 per cent of the time (satisfied, 39 per cent; dissatisfied, 71 per cent), and 76 - 100 per cent of the time (satisfied, 17 per cent; dissatisfied, 3 per cent). Whereas the original groups of satisfied and dissatisfied pharmacists were distinguishable by the percentage engaged in pharmaceutical manufacturing and in retail pharmacy, their counterparts in the validation group were not differentiated by these characteristics.

Thirteen of the 17 characteristics are equally effective in differentiating the satisfied pharmacists on the validation and standardization groups. Despite this large area of agreement there are differences that may influence our findings. Two of the 17 characteristics (both pertaining to the nature of the employing organization) differentiates the satisfied and dissatisfied pharmacists of the standardization but not of the validation group. This could stem from unreliability in our measurement of satisfaction. If it signified that the satisfied and dissatisfied members of the validation group are not as well defined as in the standardization group, then we can expect that the differentiating power of the interest scales will be underestimated.

RELIABILITY OF SCORES

The Strong Vocational Interest Blanks of the validation pharmacists were scored on each of the three experimental scales. Separate raw score totals were obtained for the odd and the even items. The coefficient of reliability of each of the three scales, computed by the odd-even technique and corrected by the Spearman-Brown formula, was: Pharmacy, .70; S-D, .69; A-B, .76. These figures are considerably lower than those reported by Strong except for his Certified Public Accountant key (r= .727), for his 36 revised scales for men had an average r of .88 as based on the records of 285 Stanford seniors. For purposes of determining reliability, the group of Stanford seniors differs from the pharmacy validation group in being larger and, presumably, in having more heterogeneous interests. Both of these factors tend to make for greater variability of scores which, in turn, increases the size of correlation coefficients (20). The coefficients obtained for the pharmacy scales are sufficiently high to justify use of the keys at least for group comparisons.

STABILITY OF ITEMS

The reliability of interest scores is related to, but not identical with, the consistency of interest keys. The coefficient of reliability refers to the degree of agreement between the scores made by individuals on the blank filled in on two separate occasions. The consistency of keys refers to the stability of the weights for the responses to each item on the blank. While the magnitude of the correlation coefficient is a by-product of item stability, it is possible for the correlation to be high and the item stability to be low. This would occur when shifts in item responses that tended to decrease scores were offset by other shifts that tended to increase scores. The respondent's likes and dislikes would thus have changed while his total interest scale scores were in close agreement.

The consistency of the weights on the three new keys, while not investigated directly, can be inferred from the interrelation of their split halves (Table 28). The odd half of the pharmacy Scale and the even half of the A-B Scale correlate about the same as the even Pharmacy and odd A-B. The odd half of the S-D Scale, however, correlates substantially higher with the even half of the Pharmacy and the A-B Scales (.71 and .34) than the even half of the S-D with the odd half of the Pharmacy and A-B Scales (.36 and .08). This discrepancy in the performance of the two halves of the S-D Scale suggests that its weights are not as stable as those of the other two scales. This becomes more apparent when the correlation coefficients computed by the odd-even technique are thought of as applying to test-retest situations. Then the S-D Scale is found to correlate more highly with the Pharmacy Scale one time than another; and the same applies to its correlations with the A-B Scale. By contrast the test-retest correlations of the Pharmacy and A-B Scales are found to be nearly alike. The instability of weights of the S-D Scale suggested by the discrepancy in the split-half correlations may result from the small size (111 dissatisfied pharmacists) of the point of reference group.

TESTS OF THE HYPOTHESES

The new scales are useful and the hypotheses of the study valid to the extent that the following propositions are true:

1. Pharmacists obtain higher scores on the Pharmacy Scales than on other scales.

2. Pharmacists make higher scores on the Pharmacy Scales than members of other occupational groups.

3. Members of other occupational groups obtain higher scores on the scale for their own occupation than they do on the Pharmacy Scales.

4. Satisfied pharmacists obtain a higher average score on the S-D Scale than on the Pharmacy Scale and the A-B Scale.

5. The difference in average scores of the satisfied and the dissatisfied is significant on the S-D Scale but not on the Pharmacy Scale or the A-B Scale.

6. Apothecary pharmacists make a higher average score on the A-B Scale than on the Pharmacy or S-D Scales.

7. The difference in average score of the apothecary and the business pharmacists is significant on the A-B Scale but not on the other two scales.

Results of the tests of these seven propositions are discussed below.

INTEROCCUPATIONAL DISCRIMINATING POWER OF THE SCALES

Proposition 1. Pharmacists obtain higher scores on the Pharmacy Scales than on other scales.

There was surprisingly little regression of the means of the total validation group toward those of the point of reference groups (men-in-general, the dissatisfied, and the business pharmacists respectively on the Pharmacy, S-D, and the A-B Scales). The mean standard scores of the criterion and validation groups, to the nearest whole number, were 48 and 46 on the Pharmacy Scale, 46 and 45 on the S-D Scale, and 44 and 45 on the A-B Scale. None of the differences was significant. In terms of interests these two total groups, standardization and validation, may be regarded as samples of the same population of pharmacists. This fact justifies comparison between the means of the validation group on the three Pharmacy Scales and the means of the standardization group on six non-pharmacy scales.

Table 13 indicates that pharmacists obtain reliably higher mean scores on their own scales than on non-pharmacy scales. It is of special interest that the differences between the pharmacists' scores on the Pharmacy Scales and on the "scientific"

Table 13

DIFFERENCE IN MEAN STANDARD SCORES OF 105 VALIDATION GROUP PHARMACISTS ON PHARMACY SCALES AND 424 STANDARDIZATION GROUP PHARMACISTS ON SIX NON-PHARMACY SCALES

Scale	Mean	Pharmacy Scale 46.285		S-D Scale 44.887		A-B Scale 45.286	
		Difference	D/σd	Difference	D/σd	Difference	D/σd
Physician	29.04	17.05	16.21	15.65	17.82	16.05	17.85
Dentist	31.08	15.21	14.28	13.81	15.43	14.21	15.50
Chemist	25.40	20.89	18.77	19.49	20.97	18.35	18.90
Office Worker	35.71	10.58	9.94	9.18	10.27	9.58	10.47
Sales Manager	35.16	11.12	10.21	9.73	10.53	10.13	10.71
Life Insurance Salesman	32.94	13.34	12.41	11.94	13.18	12.34	13.31

occupational scales (Physician, Dentist, and Chemist) are uniformly greater than the differences between the pharmacy and the business occupational scales (Office Worker, Sales Manager, and Life Insurance Salesman). The interests of pharmacists are more akin to those of office and sales workers than to those of physicians and dentists.

This appears to contradict a widely held belief that most pharmacists would prefer medicine or dentistry as an occupation and entered pharmacy as a less desirable alternative. This contradiction was apparent also when the analysis of responses on the Pharmacy Satisfaction Scale revealed that few of the dissatisfied pharmacists expressed a preference for medicine whereas many desired a business activity either in or out of pharmacy. The interpretation given to these facts is determined by one's theoretical approach to the origin, development, and stability of interests. According to Strong (65:380) and to Super (71:403) the current interest patterns of the pharmacists would probably be regarded as those present at the time they began their pharmacy training, that is, at the age range of 18 - 20. But according to Carter (5:52) and especially Bordin (4:53), with his emphasis on the dynamic nature of interests, the alleged change of interests from medicine or dentistry to pharmacy would probably be attributed to a change in the self-concept of the pharmacist resulting from a situational change. The tempering by reality of the high school senior's aspiration, according to Bordin's theory, led to the choice of pharmacy and to the adoption of the pharmaceutical occupational stereotype.

This study adds no new facts to the disagreement. Other studies like that by Kaback (33) and Remmers and Gage (44) disclose that pharmacy students' interests are more variegated than those of pharmacists, but this difference can be explained in terms of selection (the dropping out of some of the students), as well as in terms of environmental changes. It seems reasonable to believe that large numbers of pharmacists have always had lower measurable interests in medicine than in pharmacy, and that a smaller number had substantial medical interest that was reduced by their reorientation to the occupational environment.

When the letter grades made by pharmacists on the pharmacy and the non-pharmacy scales are compared (Table 14), the differentiating power of the three new scales is even more apparent.

In both comparisons, letter grades and mean standard scores, the Chemist Scale yielded scores most divergent from those of

Table 14
PERCENTAGE OF PHARMACISTS WITH A, B, AND C GRADES ON THREE PHARMACY AND SIX NON-PHARMACY SCALES[a]

Scale	Percentage with Grade of		
	A	**B**	**C**
Pharmacy	61.9	32.4	5.7
S-D	53.3	43.8	2.9
A-B	59.0	36.2	4.8
Physician	7.8	36.8	55.4
Dentist	11.6	42.7	45.7
Chemist	6.1	28.1	65.8
Office Worker	19.1	54.0	26.9
Sales Manager	18.9	51.4	29.7
Life Insurance Salesman	13.2	49.8	37.0

a. $\underline{N}$ = 105 on Pharmacy Scales and 424 on non-pharmacy.

the Pharmacy Scales. Chemists differ from dentists and physicians in that they are usually employees; their work does not require continual social stimulation; it is frequently more theoretical. Some or all of these attributes of the chemist's occupation, as they are reflected in his likes and dislikes, do not appeal to the pharmacists.

The differences in the mean scores of the pharmacists on the three Pharmacy Scales are not significant (D/σd for Pharmacy and S-D Scales = 1.16; Pharmacy and A-B = .82; A-B and S-D = .35).

These data support the hypothesis that pharmacists obtain higher scores on the three Pharmacy Scales than on the six non-pharmacy scales. The three Pharmacy Scales are about equally efficient in differentiating pharmacy from non-pharmacy interest patterns.

Proposotion 2. Pharmacists make higher scores on the Pharmacy Scales than members of other occupational groups.

Fifty-two students, 43 seniors, and 9 juniors, at the College of Medicine of Syracuse University filled in the Strong Vocational Interest Blank in 1947 as part of a study by Clendenen (7). These were scored on the Physician and on the three Pharmacy Scales.

Table 15 indicates that pharmacists score significantly higher than medical college students on the Pharmacy and the S-D Scales ($D/\sigma d$ = 6.85 and 3.85), but that the students make a mean standard score reliably higher than the pharmacists' on the A-B scale ($D/\sigma d$ = 2.84). Apparently the contrast between apothecary and business pharmacist interests brings out sharply the likes and dislikes that are characteristic of medical college upperclassmen. The A-B Scale is much more of a science scale than the Pharmacy or S-D Scales. Had this test been conducted with non-pharmacists from a non-scientific occupation it is possible that the A-B Scale would have successfully differentiated two occupational groups.

The data uphold the proposition that pharmacists make higher scores on the Pharmacy and S-D Scales than non-pharmacists. The A-B Scale, however, fails to meet this test of validity, at least with a medical non-pharmacist population.

Proposition 3. Members of other occupational groups obtain higher scores on the scale for their own occupation than they do on the Pharmacy Scales.

Table 15

MEAN STANDARD SCORES OF 105 VALIDATION GROUP PHARMACISTS AND 52 MEDICAL COLLEGE UPPERCLASSMEN ON PHARMACY SCALES

Scale	Pharmacists	Medical Upperclassmen	Difference	$D/\sigma d$
Pharmacy	46.29	35.77	10.92	6.85
S-D	44.89	40.27	4.62	3.85
A-B	45.29	48.37	-3.35	2.84

EFFECTIVENESS OF SCALES

Table 16 shows that medical college upperclassmen earn significantly higher mean standard scores on the Physician Scale than on the Pharmacy or S-D Scales ($D/\sigma d$ = 4.42 and 2.52). The mean standard score of the students on the A-B Scale was significantly higher than on the Physician ($D/\sigma d$ = 2-24).

Table 17 gives the distribution of A, B and C letter grades of the medical students on the Physician and the three Pharmacy Scales. They performed best on the A-B Scale earning more A's (73 per cent) and fewer C's (none, in fact) than on the other scales including the Physician.

Table 16

DIFFERENCES IN MEAN STANDARD SCORES OF 52
MEDICAL UPPERCLASSMEN ON PHYSICIAN
AND ON THREE PHARMACY SCALES

Scale	Mean Score	Difference from Physician	$D/\sigma d$
Physician	44.50		
Pharmacy	33.37	9.24	4.43
S-D	40.27	4.24	2.52
A-B	48.64	-4.14	2.24

Table 17

LETTER GRADES OF 52 MEDICAL UPPERCLASSMEN
ON PHYSICIAN AND PHARMACY SCALES

Scale	Percentage with Grade of		
	A	B	C
Physician	57.7	30.8	11.5
Pharmacy	11.5	61.6	26.9
S-D	23.1	73.1	3.8
A-B	73.1	26.9	

Their grades were lowest on the Pharmacy Scale in which 12 per cent had A and 27 per cent C grades. On the S- D Scale they had 23 per cent A and four per cent C grades. In contrast, they had 58 per cent A and 12 per cent C grades on their own Physician Scale.

The poor performance of the A-B Scale in rejecting medical students indicates the character of this scale in contrast with the other two. The A-B Scale is more heavily weighted with the science interests of the medical student than even the Physician Scale.

Table 18 shows that the mean standard scores of 152 satisfied apothecary pharmacists compared with those of 135 satisfied business pharmacists are consistently higher on the scientific occupational scales and lower on the business occupational scales, although only on the Chemist Scale is the difference significant. Thus, differences in interest between the two, apothecary and business pharmacists, do exist. The differences are slight when their distance from a men-in-general group is compared, because of the large area of agreement between them, but when their interests are contrasted, the differences stand out sharply enough to select persons with the scientific interests of medical students.

Table 18

STANDARD SCORES OF 152 APOTHECARY AND 135 BUSINESS SATISFIED PHARMACISTS ON SIX NON-PHARMACY SCALES

	Apothecary	Business
Physician	29.7	27.9
Dentist	31.7	29.7
Chemist	26.3	23.0
Office Worker	36.1	36.3
Sales Manager	35.2	37.4
Life Insurance Salesman	32.9	34.7

EFFECTIVENESS OF SCALES

Non-pharmacists obtain higher scores on their own scale than on two of the Pharmacy Scales, S-D and Pharmacy. Both of these, especially the Pharmacy Scale, succeed in rejecting non-pharmacists. The A-B Scale lacks this differentiating power, at least with medical college upperclassmen.

The question whether or not these medical students are members of another occupational group needs to be considered. Students who "plan to enter" an occupation do not normally make a reliable occupational group for validation purposes because of the high percentage who change their plans, or have them altered by circumstance prior to entry into the profession. This valid criticism of the use of students does not apply to a group of advanced medical college students, as their professional orientation is definite. Their average age is 23. All of them are upperclassmen, more than 80 per cent of them seniors. The attrition rate among upperclassmen in a medical college is negligible. Unless interests change materially as one changes his status from medical college upperclassman to hospital interne to practicing physician, these students are a fair sample of a non-pharmacy occupational population. Strong said that "students headed for a profession have in the main rather clear cut interests in that direction" (63:420). He reported a rank-order correlation of .91 between the interest profiles of medical students and adult physicians.

INTRA-OCCUPATIONAL DISCRIMINATING POWER OF THE SCALES:
SATISFIED AND DISSATISFIED PHARMACISTS

Proposition 4. Satisfied pharmacists obtain a higher average score on the S-D Scale than on the other two Pharmacy Scales.

Table 19 shows that satisfied pharmacists do not make a higher average on the S-D Scale than on either of the other two scales. In fact, the mean standard score is identical to that on the A-B Scale and lower than that on the Pharmacy Scale, although the latter difference is not significant ($D/\sigma d = 1.45$).

Why did the S-D Scale fail in this test of validity? The satisfied validation pharmacists scored lower than the satisfied standardization pharmacists on the Pharmacy and S-D Scales and higher on the A-B. The differences between the means of these two satisfied groups were not significant on the Pharmacy and A-B Scales ($D/\sigma d = 1.56$ and 1.43); but the difference between the satisfied validation and standardization pharmacists was

Table 19

DIFFERENCE IN MEAN STANDARD SCORES OF 71
SATISFIED PHARMACISTS ON S-D SCALE
AND OTHER PHARMACY SCALES

Scale	Mean	Difference from S-D	$D/\sigma d$
S-D	45.96		
Pharmacy	47.78	1.82	1.45
A-B	45.96		

significant on the S-D Scale ($D/\sigma d$ = 3.75). This weakness in the S-D Scale may be attributed either to an inadequacy in our sample of satisfied validation pharmacists or to a deficiency in the S-D Scale, or to both. As we found above, the satisfied pharmacists were not so different from the dissatisfied in the validation group as in the standardization group. For this reason they do not constitute as good a sample of satisfied pharmacists. On the other hand, the fact that the satisfied validation pharmacists scored approximately the same as the satisfied standardization pharmacists on the Pharmacy and A-B Scales, but significantly lower on the S-D Scale, suggests that some of the differences between the satisfied and dissatisfied members of the criterion groups that determined the weights of this key were peculiar to that sample of individuals and not characteristic of satisfied pharmacist.

Whatever the reason, the fact remains that satisfied pharmacists do not obtain a higher average score on the S-D Scale than on the other two Pharmacy Scales.

Proposition 5. The difference in mean scores of the satisfied and dissatisfied pharmacists is significant on the S-D Scale but not on the Pharmacy and A-B Scales.

When the mean standard scores of the satisfied and dissatisfied members of the criterion group were compared, the critical ratios were highly significant on the Pharmacy and S-D Scales ($D/\sigma d$ = 5.9 and 13.3). The ratio on the A-B Scale (1.6) was not reliable.

As Table 20 shows, the difference between the means of the satisfied and dissatisfied validation pharmacists on the S-D Scale was reliable ($D/\sigma d$ = 1.97), whereas the difference on the Pharmacy Scale could be accepted as valid only at the .08 level

($D/\sigma d$ = 1.83). The difference was not significant on the A-B Scale ($D/\sigma d$ = 1.47).

Comparison of the percentage of A letter grades earned by the satisfied and dissatisfied on the three scales shows no significant differences (Table 21). When the percentages of combined A and B plus grades were compared, the S-D Scale was the only one that succeeded in differentiating the two by a significant margin. Among the satisfied, 87 per cent earned one of the two top letter grades compared with only 59 per cent of the dissatisfied ($D/\sigma d$ = 2.93).

The scores of the satisfied and dissatisfied pharmacists of the standardization group on the six non-pharmacy scales were compared in the belief they would shed some light on the nature of pharmacy satisfaction. The dissatisfied pharmacists averaged higher scores than the satisfied on each of the three scientific non-pharmacy occupational scales (Table 22), but none of the differences is reliable. On two of the business occupational scales, however, the satisfied pharmacists made reliably higher mean scores. Two of the non-pharmacy scales, Sales manager and Life Insurance Salesman, differentiated the satisfied and the dissatisfied groups ($D/\sigma d$ = 3.73, 2.73) more effectively than the S-D Scale did with the validation pharmacists. In accomplishing this, however, the Sales Manager Scale, for example, selected only 35 per cent of the satisfied pharmacists (A and B plus scores) in contrast with the 87 percent selected by the S-D Scale. The Office Worker Scale did not successfully differentiate the two satisfaction groups.

Table 20

DIFFERENCE BETWEEN 71 SATISFIED AND 32 DISSATISFIED VALIDATION-GROUP PHARMACISTS ON THREE PHARMACY SCALES

Scale	Satisfied	Dissatisfied	Difference	$D/\sigma d$
Pharmacy	47.78	43.66	4.12	1.83
S-D	45.96	42.34	3.61	1.97
A-B	45.96	43.56	2.40	1.47

Table 21

DIFFERENCE BETWEEN 71 SATISFIED AND 32 DISSATISFIED VALIDATION-GROUP IN PERCENTAGE OF A AND OF COMBINED A AND B+ LETTER GRADES

Percentage with letter Grade of

Scale	A					A or B+		
	Satisfied	Dissatisfied	Difference	D/σd	Satisfied	Dissatisfied	Difference	D/σd
Phar-macy	66.20	56.24	9.96	.96	80.28	68.74	11.54	1.22
S-D	57.75	43.75	14.00	1.33	87.33	59.38	27.95	2.93
A-B	61.97	50.00	11.97	1.14	78.87	78.12	-00.75	

Table 22
COMPARISON OF 313 SATISFIED AND 111 DISSATISFIED STANDARDIZATION-GROUP ON SIX NON-PHARMACY SCALES

Scale	Satisfied	Dissatisfied	Difference	D/σd
Physician	28.65	30.38	1.73	1.45
Dentist	30.50	31.87	1.37	1.11
Chemist	24.83	27.05	2.21	1.57
Office Worker	36.19	34.34	1.84	1.74
Sales Manager	36.32	31.91	4.40	3.73
Life Insurance Salesman	33.79	30.56	3.23	2.73

The disparity between business and scientific occupational interest is not so great for the dissatisfied (average of 32 and 30 standard scores) as it is for the satisfied (35 and 28). Another difference between the two is in the type of business interest that is stressed. The satisfied pharmacists average as high on the Sales Manager as on the Office Worker Scale, whereas the predominant vocational interest of the dissatisfied is that of the Office Worker. This may reflect the desire expressed by several dissatisfied pharmacists for jobs involving little direct contact with the public.

In summary, the S-D Scale shows its superiority over the other scales in its successful differentiation of the satisfied and the dissatisfied. The Pharmacy Scale produces a fairly large but not reliable difference between the two. When combined A and B plus scores of the satisfied and dissatisfied are compared for the three scales, the S-D Scale shows marked superiority. Two business non-pharmacy scales differentiate the satisfied and dissatisfied better even than the S-D Scale, but in doing so they reject a majority of the satisfied pharmacists.

The proposition that the difference between the satisfied and the dissatisfied on the S-D Scale is more significant than on the other two is supported by this evidence.

INTRA-OCCUPATIONAL DISCRIMINATING POWER OF THE SCALES: APOTHECARY AND BUSINESS PHARMACISTS

Proposition 6. Apothecary pharmacists obtain a higher average score on the A-B Scale than on the Pharmacy or S-D Scales.

The apothecary pharmacists made a slightly higher mean score on the Pharmacy Scale than on the A-B (Table 23), but the difference between the two means was far from significant ($D/\sigma d$ = .19). They scored higher on the A-B than on the S-D scale, but this difference, though larger, was also unreliable ($D/\sigma d$ = .85).

The 188 apothecary criterion pharmacists had a mean standard score of 49.5 as compared with the score of 46.7 of the 49 apothecaries in the validation group. The difference is significant ($D/\sigma d$ = 2.10).

The hypothesis that apothecary pharmacists obtain a higher average score on the A-B than on the other scales is not substantiated. In an earlier discussion on the apothecary and business pharmacists in the criterion group, it was noted that the apothecary group consisted of a reliably higher percentage of the satisfied than did the business group.

Table 23

DIFFERENCE IN MEAN STANDARD SCORE OF 49 APOTHECARY PHARMACISTS ON A-B AND OTHER PHARMACY SCALES

Scale	Mean	Difference from A-B	$D/\sigma d$
A-B	46.67		
Pharmacy	46.98	-.31	.19
S-D	45.33	1.34	.85

This relationship is likewise true of the validation group. Further analysis disclosed that the differences in the percentage of satisfied pharmacists between the criterion and validation apothecaries, and between the criterion and validation business pharmacists, were not significant. The difference in mean scores of the criterion and validation apothecaries was reliable. It appears that the failure of the A-B Scale to differentiate apothecary and business pharmacists reflects basic defects in the scale (due perhaps to the system of classifying the two criterion groups) rather than in the validation sample.

Proposition 7. The difference in average score of the apothecary and the business pharmacists is significant on the A-B Scale but not on the other two.

In Table 24 are shown the differences in the mean scores of the apothecary and the business pharmacists on the three scales. None of them is significant. The critical ratio of the means is larger on the A-B Scale ($D/\sigma d = 1.51$) than on the others, but this too falls short of reliability.

In a further test of the comparative discriminating power of the three scales critical ratios of the percentages of A letter grades of apothecary and business pharmacists were computed (Table 25). The difference of 11 per cent on the A-B Scale was the largest, but this was not significant ($D/\sigma d = 1.12$).

When the percentages of combined A and B, plus grades of apothecaries and business pharmacists on the three scales were computed, differences on the Pharmacy and S-D Scales were negligible, and the difference of 4.5 per cent on the A-B Scale was not reliable ($D/\sigma d = .55$).

Table 24

DIFFERENCE BETWEEN APOTHECARY AND BUSINESS PHARMACISTS ON THREE PHARMACY SCALES

Scale	Apothecary	Business	Difference	$D/\sigma d$
Pharmacy	46.98	46.69	0.29	0.16
S-D	45.33	45.06	0.27	0.18
A-B	46.67	44.25	2.42	1.51

Table 25

DIFFERENCE BETWEEN 49 APOTHECARY AND 48 BUSINESS PHARMACISTS IN PERCENTAGES OF A, AND OF COMBINED A AND B+ LETTER GRADES

Percentage with letter Grade of

Scale	A				A or B+			
	Apothecary	Business	Difference	D/σd	Apothecary	Business	Difference	D/σd
Pharmacy	63.3	66.7	-3.4	0.35	77.6	78.2	-0.6	
S-D	57.2	52.1	5.1	0.51	79.6	81.2	-1.6	.20
A-B	65.3	54.2	11.1	1.12	81.6	77.1	4.5	.55

EFFECTIVENESS OF SCALES

It was pointed out above that the difference in interests between apothecary and business pharmacists was large enough to weight a scale that selects medical students successfully. Why then does it not differentiate between apothecary and business pharmacists? Presumably, the major difference that exists between the two groups is in terms of scientific interest, and it is probable that only those at the extremes of the two groups were sufficiently different to account for the weights. The lack of differentiation between the two on the A-B Scale probably reflects the true lack of difference between them and suggests that most pharmacists, in interest as in actual practice, are both apothecary and business pharmacists.

Although the A-B Scale selects apothecary and rejects business pharmacists with slightly more success than the other scales, the difference is not significant. The hypothesis that the A-B Scale differentiates apothecary and business pharmacists better than the other two has not been validated.

VII Interrelationship and Evaluation of Scales

OUR tests of the seven propositions of this investigation have suggested a degree of relationship among the three scales, especially between the Pharmacy and the S-D Scales. The total validation group averaged approximately the same on the three scales. The disparity between the scores of pharmacists on each of the Pharmacy Scales and on six non-pharmacy scales was similar in each case. Both the Pharmacy and the S-D Scales rejected non-pharmacists successfully. Neither the satisfied pharmacists nor the apothecary pharmacists averaged significantly higher, or earned a reliably higher percentage of A letter grades on one scale than on the other.

There were also a few indications that the scales are not identical. The non-pharmacists scored reliably higher than the pharmacists on the A-B Scale; likewise, they scored significantly higher on the A-B Scale and lower on the Pharmacy and S-D Scales than on the Physician Scale. The S-D Scale, unlike the other two, and especially unlike the A-B Scale, reliably differentiated the satisfied and the dissatisfied pharmacists.

INTERRELATION OF THE THREE INTEREST SCALES

The intercorrelations of standard scores of the validation pharmacists on the three scales are given in Table 26. There is a negligible relationship between the A-B and the Pharmacy scales ($r = -.15$) and between the A-B and the S-D scales ($r = .14$). These correlations are not significant.

Table 26

INTERCORRELATIONS OF SCORES OF 105 VALIDATION-GROUP PHARMACISTS ON THREE PHARMACY SCALES

Scale	Pharmacy	S-D
S-D	.57[a]	
A-B	-.15	.14

a. When $N = 105$, r must exceed .193 for significance at the .05 level (20:299).

A substantial relationship between the Pharmacy Scale and the S-D Scale (r= .57) was to be expected in view of the fact that the scales differ only in respect to the point of reference used (men-in-general on the Pharmacy; the dissatisfied on the S-D). Nevertheless, the correlation between the two is not so large as the reliability coefficient of either of the scales.

Correlations of the standard scores of the satisfied validation pharmacists on the three scales are shown in Table 27. The r of .34, much smaller than the total group correlation between the Pharmacy and the S-D Scales, is significant. The relationship between the A-B and S-D Scales is now even more negligible, and the disparity between the Pharmacy and the A-B Scales more marked than with the total groups. The Pharmacy A-B correlation (r= -.31) shows a significant negative relationship. Thus the scores of satisfied pharmacists on the Pharmacy Scale tend to be positively related to their scores on the S-D Scale and negatively related to those on the A-B, suggesting that the typical satisfied pharmacist, as well as the typical pharmacist, is a businessman. When applied to satisfied pharmacists the three scales are less alike than when used with all pharmacists of the validation group, probably because of the restricted range of the sample of satisfied pharmacists.

Table 27

INTERCORRELATIONS OF SCORES OF 71 SATISFIED VALIDATION-GROUP PHARMACISTS ON THREE PHARMACY SCALES

Scale	Pharmacy	S-D
S-D	.34[a]	
A-B	-.31	.08

a. When N=71, r must exceed .234 for significance at the .05 level (20:299).

INTER-HALF-SCALE CORRELATIONS

As a further check on the overlapping as well as on the reliability of the scales, inter-half-scale correlations were computed; that is, the odd half of each scale was matched with the even of each of the other two, and the even with the odds (Table 28). Except for the correlation between odd S-D and even Pharmacy (r= .71), all of the cross-scale r's are substantially lower than the reliability coefficients of the scales. In other words, the odd half of each scale is more like its even half than like the even half of another scale. The odd S-D and the even Pharmacy Scales correlate more highly (.71) than either does with the opposite half of its own scale (.70; .69). The odd S-D and the even A-B are more highly correlated (.34) than the even S-D and the odd A-B (.-08).

Both halves of the Pharmacy Scale are correlated significantly with their opposite halves on the S-D Scale. The negative correlations between the even Pharmacy and odd A-B, and the odd Pharmacy and even A-B, are reliable. Correlation between the odd S-D and even A-B Scales is reliable, while the even S-D and odd A-B relationship is insignificant.

As discussed above, these split-half intercorrelations raise some doubt about the stability of item responses on the S-D Scale. While the two halves of the S-D Scale have a fairly high correlation coefficient (suggesting reliability of scores), the odd half is much more like the other two scales than is the even half (suggesting item inconsistency).

Table 28

ODD-EVEN HALF-SCALE CORRELATIONS [a] OF SCORES OF 105 VALIDATION-GROUP PHARMACISTS WITHIN AND BETWEEN THREE PHARMACY SCALES

Scale	Even Pharmacy	Even S-D	Even A-B
Odd Pharmacy	.70[b]	.36	-.24
Odd S-D	.71	.69	.34
Odd A-B	-.29	-.08	.76

a. Corrected by Spearman-Brown formula.
b. r must exceed .193 for significance at the .05 level.

RELATION BETWEEN INTEREST AND SATISFACTION

In order to determine the relationship between feeling of satisfaction as measured by the Pharmacy Satisfaction Scale, and interest in pharmacy, correlations were computed between the index of satisfaction and standard score on each of the three scales. As shown in Table 29 the satisfaction index correlates approximately the same with the Pharmacy and S-D Scales (r = .30 and .27). These correlations, both of them significant, imply that a small but positive relationship exists between scores on the Pharmacy or S-D Scale for the Strong Vocational Interest Blank and the job satisfaction of the pharmacists. The correlation with the A-B Scale was unreliable.

EVALUATION OF THE FINDINGS

The correlation between Pharmacy and S-D Scales was high, almost as high as the odd-even correlation of each scale. Unless the S-D Scale performs the function of selecting pharmacists and rejecting non-pharmacists more effectively than the Pharmacy Scale, or unless it performs some other unique function, it is superfluous. And if this is so, utilization of the dissatisfied instead of men-in-general as the point of reference in construction of the scale has no purpose.

Table 29

CORRELATIONS OF INDEX OF SATISFACTION ON PHARMACY SATISFACTION SCALE AND OF STANDARD SCORE ON THREE PHARMACY INTEREST SCALES, FOR 103 VALIDATION-GROUP PHARMACISTS [a]

Scale	r With Index of Satisfaction
Pharmacy	.30 [b]
S-D	.27
A-B	.11

a. Two of the 105 validation-group pharmacists were unclassified as to satisfaction.

b. When N = 103, r must exceed .190 for significance at the .05 level (20:299).

Effectiveness of The New Point of Reference

The S-D Scale did perform almost as effectively as the Pharmacy Scale in selecting pharmacists and rejecting non-pharmacists. In addition, the S-D Scale did what neither of the others accomplished: (1) it distinguished between the satisfied and the dissatisfied when mean scores were compared; (2) it differentiated between the satisfied and dissatisfied in a comparison of percentages receiving A and B plus grades. Within the limits of confidence that can be placed in a scale that is based on a comparison of only 313 satisfied and 111 dissatisfied pharmacists, the S-D Scale must be regarded as a more effective instrument for the differentation of the satisfied and dissatisfied members of pharmacy than the other two scales.

The S-D Scale demonstrated this superiority over the Pharmacy Scale despite the fact that the Pharmacy Scale, unlike other Strong vocational interest scales, was built upon a criterion group of satisfied pharmacists. The only difference between these two scales is in the point of reference. The success of the S-D Scale in differentiating the satisfied and dissatisfied must be attributed to the use of the dissatisfied pharmacists as the point of reference. There is reason to believe that if the S-D Scale were compared with a pharmacy scale constructed in the usual manner, in which no deliberate effort was made to exclude the dissatisfied from the criterion group, the S-D Scale would show more marked superiority. For example, on the A-B Scale, which is only partially contaminated with satisfaction (because of the high percentage of satisfied apothecary pharmacists), the satisfied pharmacists have less than one per cent more A and B plus grades than the dissatisfied. The differences on the Pharmacy and the S-D Scales are 12 and 28 per cent respectively.

Several other considerations add further weight to the validating data. There is some question concerning the representativeness of the sample of satisfied validation pharmacists, who were more like the dissatisfied in their group than was true of the criterion group. They were differentiated from the dissatisfied by two less characteristics (out of 17) than were the satisfied and dissatisfied criterion pharmacists.

It has been pointed out that our dissatisfied pharmacists were only relatively dissatisfied. A very sizable proportion of both satisfied and dissatisfied criterion pharmacists were borderline cases. A majority of the dissatisfied were glad they were pharmacists. The use of two extreme satisfaction groups, for weight, norm, and validation purposes, would lead to sharper delineation of interests.[1] It would very probably increase the relationship of feeling of satisfaction and interest score. Probably it would also decrease the relationship between the Pharmacy and the S-D Scale, which is suggested by the decline in the correlation between the two when only satisfied pharmacists' scores are compared. To what extent this correlation could be reduced is difficult to estimate. Some overlapping must be expected as representing a true area of agreement in interest of men-in-general and dissatisfied pharmacists, the two points of reference.

Stability of Pharmacy Satisfaction

The value of this or any improved scale of this type will depend in part on its reliability. The reliability coefficient of an inventory based on satisfaction cannot be accepted with confidence unless its criterion groups are stable. This investigation has given us no information on the stability of pharmacy satisfaction. From comments written on the Pharmacy Satisfaction Scales some of the men can be regarded as having immutable attitudes toward pharmacy, but a high percentage of the dissatisfied criticized certain conditions within pharmacy rather than the more basic professional activities.

A high percentage of the dissatisfied pharmacists criticized the length of the work week. We may ask what effect a change in the length of the work week would have upon their satisfaction in pharmacy. If it will then make them satisfied pharmacists, will it also give them "satisfied interests"? As mentioned previously several studies (33, 44) indicate that the interests of pharmacy students are different from those of pharmacists. Two interpretations can be made: (1) that the interests of pharmacy students are modified during their early professional years under the impact of new experience; (2) that a process of selection eliminates those students whose interests differ widely from pharmacy interests. If interest measurement is to be linked with job satisfaction it is important to determine the effects of changed conditions upon the feeling of satisfaction. It will be necessary to know whether changes in working

---

[1]. In this study it was impossible to use only the two extreme groups. When interest scales are to be established, it is essential to utilize every available return unless the number exceeds 500.

conditions, e.g., length of work week, will bring about a fundamental alteration in the pattern of interests. The evidence thus far indicates that the interests are not changed (63, 70. 71), but further investigation like that proposed by Bordin (4) is needed.

Failure to Differentiate Apothecary and Business Interest

The A-B Scale does not correlate significantly with either of the other scales, except for a negative correlation (-.31) with the Pharmacy Scale for satisfied pharmacists. Presumably the A-B Scale measures something other than the Pharmacy and S-D Scales. It serves about as well as the others in selecting pharmacists, but it fails to exclude non-pharmacists whose interests are scientific. This scale is unsuccessful in the most significant test of validity in that it fails to perform the function for which it was designed, namely, the separation of apothecary and business pharmacists.

While there is evidence that the groups of apothecary and satisfied pharmacists overlap a great deal (84 per cent of the apothecaries are satisfied in contrast to 59 per cent of the business pharmacists) when standard scores of satisfied pharmacists are intercorrelated, the A-B Scale works even more unlike the other two, becoming less like the S-D Scale and more unlike the Pharmacy Scale. A man was classified as an apothecary if he reported devoting more than 25 per cent of his time to prescription work, providing he did not voluntarily complain this was excessive or unpleasant. In other words, the man had to be either a satisfied pharmacist, or a dissatisfied pharmacist who was not dissatisfied with his prescription work, to be classified as an apothecary. The error in this technique of classification is that the apothecary pharmacist may be satisfied not because of the apothecary work but because his primary business interests have an outlet during the remaining 74 per cent or less of his time, whether from the management of his business, the purchase of new stock, or the frequent customer contact which even most apothecary pharmacists experience. Such a pharmacist's satisfaction emanates more from his business activities than from the apothecary, and his attitudes and interests are those of the business pharmacist.

Most of the apothecary pharmacists in this study devoted 26 - 75 per cent of their time to prescription. Most of them, that is, spend at least 25 per cent of their time on business activities. It is very likely that our sample of apothecary pharmacists includes men who spend 50 per cent of their time in prescription work, 50 per cent in business activities, who enjoy the business aspects more than the apothecary, and who, because of the business activities, are very well satisfied in pharmacy. Personal interviews with pharmacists disclosed that a substantial number of them prefer the combination of functions.

Despite the fact that we have failed to differentiate the interests of the two groups, there are some cues suggesting that differences may exist (Table 18). In so far as they exist we have failed in this study to translate them into an effective interest scale. Further efforts in this direction should seek first a more valid method for identifying the two groups. When this is accomplished, it is likely that the pharmacy profession will be found to consist of two small minority groups (apothecary and business) and a large majority group belonging in neither of the pure, extreme groups.

VIII Summary and Conclusions

THE purpose of this study was to answer several questions about the significance of job satisfaction data to interest measurement. It was decided to use pharmacists as subjects in the investigation which would seek answers to the following questions:

1. By excluding the dissatisfied members of an occupation, can an interest scale be developed which will differentiate the satisfied from the dissatisfied in this occupation?

2. Will the dissatisfied members of an occupation serve as a better point of reference than a group of men-in-general in constructing an interest scale for the differentiation of the satisfied?

3. Do the interests of pharmacists form a pattern distinguishable from those of other occupations?

4. Can the pharmacists who devote less than 25 per cent of their time to prescription work or research be differentiated by their interests from the apothecary pharmacists who devote more than 25 per cent of their time to the scientific activities of the profession?

Strong Vocational Interest Blanks and Pharmacy Satisfaction Scales were sent to 1500 randomly selected pharmacists in New York State (except New York City). The 450 usable returns were subdivided into 333 satisfied, 117 dissatisfied; 188 apothecary and 194 business pharmacists. Characteristics differentiating the satisfied and dissatisfied pharmacists were found (Table 4).

Three scales were constructed (Table 10): the Vocational Interest Scale for Pharmacists (Pharmacy Scale), in which satisfied pharmacists are contrasted with men-in-general; the Satisfied vs. Dissatisfied Pharmacists Scale (S-D-Scale), in which satisfied are contrasted with dissatisfied pharmacists; the Apothecary vs. Business Pharmacists Scale (A-B Scale), in which apothecary pharmacists (26 - 100 per cent of work time devoted to prescription work) are contrasted with business pharmacists (no more than 25 per cent of time given to prescription work).

The 105 validation pharmacists, (71 satisfied, 32 dissatisfied; 49 apothecary, 48 business), most of them from Connecticut and

SUMMARY AND CONCLUSIONS

New York, were scored on the scales. The scales were found to be sufficiently reliable for group use (Table 28).

Seven propositions were formulated to test the validity of the scales and thereby of the hypotheses. They are rewritten below in the form of conclusions conforming with the findings of the study.

1. Pharmacists obtain higher scores on the Pharmacy Scales than on other scales (Tables 13 and 14).

2. They make higher scores on the Pharmacy and the S-D Scales than non-pharmacists. The A-B Scale, however, fails to meet this test of validity with a medical non-pharmacist population (Table 15).

3. Non-pharmacists earn higher scores on the scale for their own occupation than they do on the Pharmacy and S-D Scales. The A-B Scale, however, lacks this differentiating power for a medical non-pharmacist population (Tables 16 and 17).

4. Satisfied pharmacists do not make a higher average score on the S-D than on the other two Pharmacy Scales (Table 19).

5. The difference between the satisfied and dissatisfied pharmacists in mean standard score and in combined A and B plus grades is significant on the S-D Scale but falls short of significance on the Pharmacy and A-B Scales (Tables 20 and 21).

6. Apothecary pharmacists do not obtain a higher average score on the A-B than on the other scales (Table 23).

7. The difference in average scores of the apothecary and the business pharmacists is not significant on the A-B Scale or on the other scales (Tables 24 and 25).

The Pharmacy and the S-D Scales were found to have a fairly high relationship (Table 26), particularly the odd half of the S-D and the even half of the Pharmacy Scales (Table 28). The S-D and the A-B Scales showed very little relationship. The A-B and Pharmacy Scales were negatively related. The split-half intercorrelations of the three scales point to the possible instability of item responses on the S-D Scale.

Both the Pharmacy and the S-D Scales were significantly related to the feeling of satisfaction of the pharmacists as measured by the Pharmacy Satisfaction Scale (Table 29).

The findings of this investigation may be summarized as follows:

SUMMARY AND CONCLUSIONS

1. Members of the pharmacy profession have a recognizable pattern of likes and dislikes.

2. Pharmacists have been successfully differentiated from other occupational groups on two new pharmacy scales of the Strong Vocational Interest Blank, one of which (Pharmacy Scale) employed Strong's men-in-general group as point of reference, and the other (S-D Scale), a group of dissatisfied pharmacists. In construction of both scales the criterion groups were satisfied pharmacists.

3. A vocational interest scale (S-D Scale) of the Strong Vocational Interest Blank has been developed which differentiates groups of satisfied and dissatisfied pharmacists with moderate success.

4. The exclusion of the dissatisfied pharmacists from the weight group was not sufficient to accomplish this, for the Pharmacy Scale did not differentiate the two successfully. The S-D and Pharmacy Scales differ only in respect to the point of reference. To this alone, therefore, must the variance in the differentiating ability of the two scales be attributed.

5. Both scales in which the criterion groups were limited to satisfied pharmacists were significantly correlated with the feeling of satisfaction.

6. There is some evidence of a difference in the interests of apothecary and business pharmacists, but these differences were not sufficiently great to be converted into a differentiating scale (A-B Scale) by the methods used.

7. The reliability coefficients, lower than the average for all of Strong's scales, are sufficiently high to justify use of the keys at least for group comparisons. The greater homogeneity and smaller size of the groups used to determine reliability in this study probably account for the lower coefficients. The smallness of the point of reference group of the S-D Scale (111 dissatisfied pharmacists) is a possible cause for the implied instability of weights.

8. Interrelationship of scores of pharmacists on the pharmacy and non-pharmacy scales suggests that the typical pharmacist, as well as the typical satisfied pharmacist, has interests similar to those of the businessman.

SUMMARY AND CONCLUSIONS

The following recommendations are made for further study in this area:

The sample. Only those members of an occupation who are at the two extremes of the continuum of satisfaction (or the continuum of job specialization in an occupation) should be used to construct the interest scale. To make this possible the occupational sample used for selection of the extreme groups should be substantially larger than in this study. It should be sufficiently large that the number of extremely dissatisfied constituting the point of reference group will provide stable weights.

The interest scales. To explore further the advantages of various criteria (e.g., membership in occupation, satisfaction) in the selection of standardization groups, and of the reference point groups (e.g., men-in-general, dissatisfied), the following types of scales might be compared: satisfied vs. dissatisfied with satisfied vs. men-in-general; satisfied vs. men-in-general with members of an occupation vs. men-in-general; members of an occupation vs. men-in-general with members of an occupation vs. dissatisfied.

Interest and satisfaction. If interest scales are to be weighted in terms of differences between the satisfied and dissatisfied members of an occupation, the relationship between change in feeling of satisfaction and the stability of interests will have to be investigated. The need exists for further research on the dynamics of interest development and job satisfaction, research that examines the social, economic, and psychological factors that interrelate to form attitudes toward self, occupations and other relevant aspects of the individual's phenomenal field.

Appendix

A STUDY OF THE INTERESTS OF SATISFIED AND DISSATISFIED PHARMACISTS

MILTON SCHWEBEL, M.A.
(ASS'T. PROFESSOR OF PSYCHOLOGY)
MOHAWK COLLEGE
ASSOCIATED COLLEGES OF UPPER NEW YORK
UTICA, NEW YORK

ENDORSERS

DEAN CHARLES W. BALLARD
  COLLEGE OF PHARMACY
  COLUMBIA UNIVERSITY
DEAN A. B. LEMON
  SCHOOL OF PHARMACY
  UNIVERSITY OF BUFFALO
DEAN FRANCIS J. O'BRIEN
  ALBANY COLLEGE OF PHARMACY
  UNION UNIVERSITY
DR. CURT P. WIMMER
  PUBLIC RELATIONS DIRECTOR
  N. Y. STATE PHARMACEUTICAL ASSOC.

ADVISORY COMMITTEE
COLUMBIA UNIVERSITY

DR. DONALD E. SUPER, CHAIRMAN
  ASSOCIATE PROFESSOR OF EDUCATION
DR. IRVING LORGE
  PROFESSOR OF EDUCATION
  EXECUTIVE OFFICER,
  INSTITUTE OF PSYCHOLOGICAL RESEARCH
DR. LAURANCE F. SHAFFER
  PROFESSOR OF EDUCATION
  HEAD, DEPARTMENT OF GUIDANCE

Dear Sir:

You are a member of a profession which does not have the advantage of special interest tests for its candidates. The medical, dental and other professions have such tests so that applicants for admission to training for their professions can be advised by the results of such procedures.

Your profession can develop an interest test which could be used as a basis for guiding young men toward or away from Pharmacy. The Strong Vocational Interest Blank could be adapted to such a purpose if adequate data were available. You are one of a group of selected Pharmacists whose help would make available such a guiding interest test.

Enclosed are a Vocational Interest Blank and a Pharmacy Satisfaction Scale (stapled to the Blank). If you will answer all of the questions, it will be possible to estimate the interest of Pharmacists.

Your responses will be considered confidential. Please do not write your name on the Interest Blank or the Scale. Simply mark your answers--your immediate reactions are best--and mail the two scales in the enclosed, stamped, self-addressed envelope.

You will be informed of the project in a forthcoming issue of the New York Pharmacist. Your cooperation will help greatly the Pharmacy Profession.

Sincerely yours,

Milton Schwebel

Enc: Vocational Interest Blank
     Pharmacy Satisfaction Scale
     Self-addressed Envelope

PHARMACY SATISFACTION SCALE

Age (last birthday) .... Sex .... Veteran of World War II? Yes ☐ No ☐ Was any member of your family in Pharmacy when you entered the profession? Yes ☐ No ☐ If so, what relationship? (e.g. uncle) ....

Name of community in which you are engaged in Pharmacy ....

Number of years of paid experience in Pharmacy .... years.

Occupation in Pharmacy (check only one box):
Owner (individual or partner) ☐   Member of corporation ☐   Employee ☐

Nature of organization owned or employed in:
Retail Pharmacy ☐   (if so, is it a chain store? Yes ☐   No ☐)
Wholesale Pharmacy ☐   Pharmacy manufacturing ☐   Hospital or other institution ☐

Percentage of time devoted to prescription or research work (in contrast with sales or management) (check only one box): 0 to 25% ☐, 26 to 75% ☐, 76 to 100% ☐

A—Place a check mark (√) in front of the statement that expresses your feelings:

.... I am glad that I am a Pharmacist.
.... I am sorry that I am a Pharmacist.

D—Check one of the following to show HOW MUCH OF THE TIME you feel satisfied with being a Pharmacist:

.... All of the time.
.... Most of the time.
.... A good deal of the time.
.... About half of the time.

APPENDIX

B—Choose the one of the following statements which best tells how you like being a Pharmacist. Place a check mark (√) in front of the statement:

.... I hate it.
.... I dislike it.
.... On the whole I don't like it.
.... I am indifferent to it.
.... I like it a little.
.... I like it fairly well.
.... On the whole I like it.
.... I like it a good deal.
.... I like it very much.
.... I am enthusiastic about it.
.... I love it.

C—Check one of the following to show how you think you compare with other people:

.... No one likes his work better than I like mine.
.... I like my work much better than most people like theirs.
.... I like my work better than most people like theirs.
.... I like my work about as well as most people like theirs.
.... I do not know how I compare with other people.
.... I dislike my work more than most people dislike theirs.
.... I dislike my work much more than most people dislike theirs.
.... No one dislikes his work more than I dislike mine.

.... Occasionally.
.... Seldom.
.... Never.

E—Check one of the following which best tells how you feel about changing your field of Pharmacy:

.... I would quit Pharmacy at once if I could get anything else to do.
.... I would take almost any other field in which I could earn as much as I am earning now.
.... I would like to leave the field of Pharmacy altogether.
.... I would like to remain a Pharmacist and change my line of work in Pharmacy.
.... I would like to change my present job for another job in Pharmacy in the same line of work.
.... I am not eager to give up Pharmacy but I would do so if I could get into a better field.
.... I cannot think of any field of work for which I would give up Pharmacy.
.... I would not exchange Pharmacy for any other field.

F—If you desire a change, state below what type of work or business or employer you prefer. (This might be a change in your line of work within Pharmacy or a change from Pharmacy to another field).

....

....

Bibliography

1. Bellows, R. M. "The Status of Selection and Counseling Techniques for Dental Students." Journal of Consulting Psychology, IV (January - February 1940), 10 - 15.
2. Benge, E. J., and D. F. Copell. "Employee Morale Survey." Modern Management, XII (January 1947), 19 - 22.
3. Berman, I. R., J. G. Darley, and D. G. Paterson. Vocational Interest Scales, Bulletin of the Employment Stabilization Research Institute, Minneapolis: University of Minnesota, III, No. 5 (1934).
4. Bordin, E. S. "A Theory of Vocational Interests as Dynamic Phenomena." Educational Psychological Measurement, III (Spring, 1943), 49 - 66.
5. Carter, H. D. "The Development of Vocational Interests." Journal of Consulting Psychology, IV (September - October, 1940), 185 - 191.
6. -----. Vocational Interests and Job Orientation. Stanford University: Stanford University Press, 1944.
7. Clendenen, D. The Relation of Certain Factors to Success in the College of Medicine of Syracuse University. Unpublished doctoral dissertation, Syracuse University, 1948.
8. Darley, J. G. "A Preliminary Study of Relations between Attitude, Adjustment and Vocational Interest Tests." Journal of Educational Psychology, XXIX (September, 1938), 467 - 473.
9. -----. Clinical Aspects and Interpretation of the Strong Vocational Interest Blank. New York: Psychological Corp., 1941.
10. -----. "Evaluation of Interest Tests." In O. J. Kaplan (ed.), Encyclopedia of Vocational Guidance, I, 621 - 626. New York: Philosophical Library, 1948.
11. Dickson, W. J. "The Hawthorne Plan of Personnel Counseling." American Journal of Orthopsychiatry, XV (April, 1945), 343 - 347.
12. Ellis, A., and J. R. Gerberich. "Interests and Attitudes." Review of Educational Research, XVII (February, 1947), 64 - 77.
13. Estes, S. G., and D. Horn. "Interest Patterns as Related to Fields of Concentration among Engineering Students." Journal of Psychology, VII (January, 1939), 29 - 36.

14. Fisher, R. A., and F. Yates. Statistical Tables for Biological, Agricultural and Medical Research. London: Oliver and Boyd, 1938.
15. Fisher, V. E., and J. V. Hanna. The Dissatisfied Worker. New York: MacMillan, 1931.
16. Frendsen, A. "Appraisal of Interests in Guidance." Journal of Educational Research, XXXIX (September, 1945), 1 - 12.
17. Fryer, D. The Measurement of Interests. New York: Henry Holt and Co., 1931.
18. -----. "Validating Measures of Interest, with Particular Reference to Group Interest Scales." Personnel Journal, XI (August, 1932), 103 - 110.
19. Fuller, S. E. "Goodyear Aircraft Employee Counseling." Personnel Journal, XXIII (October, 1944), 145 - 153.
20. Garrett, H. E. Statistics in Psychology and Education. New York: Longmans, Green and Co., 1947.
21. Habbe, S. "Job Attitudes of Life Insurance Agents." Journal of Applied Psychology, XXXI (April, 1947), 111 - 118.
22. Hahn, M. E., and C. I. Williams. "The Measured Interests of Marine Corps Women Reservists." Journal of Applied Psychology, XXIX (June, 1945), 198 - 211.
23. Hand, T. "Job Satisfaction." In O. J. Kaplan (ed.), Encyclopedia of Vocational Guidance, I, 668 - 675. New York: Philosophical Library, 1948.
24. Hand, T., R. Hoppock, and P. Zlatchin. "Job Satisfaction: Researches of 1944 - 1945." Occupations, XXVI (April, 1948), 425 - 431.
25. Hoppock, R. Job Satisfaction. New York: Harper and Brothers, 1935.
26. -----. "Age and Job Satisfaction." Psychological Monograph, XLVII (1936), 115 - 118.
27. Hoppock, R., and T. Hand. "Job Satisfaction Researches of 1942 - 1943." Occupations, XXIII (April, 1945), 412 - 415.
28. Hoppock, R., and C. Odom. "Job Satisfaction--Researches and Opinions of 1938 - 1939." Occupations, XIX (October, 1940), 24 - 28.
29. Hoppock, R., H. A. Robinson, and P. Zlatchin. "Job Satisfaction Researches of 1946 - 1947." Occupations, XXVII (December, 1948), 167 - 175.

BIBLIOGRAPHY

30. Hoppock, R., and R. H. Shaffer. "Job Satisfaction--Researches and Opinions of 1940 - 1941." Occupations, XXI (February, 1943), 457 - 463.
31. Hoppock, R., and S. Spiegler. "Job Satisfaction Researches of 1935 - 1937." Occupations, XVI (April, 1938), 636-643.
32. Hoppock, R., and D. E. Super. "Vocational and Educational Satisfaction." In D. Fryer and E. R. Henny (eds.), Psychotechnology and Psychological Practice, New York: Farrar and Rinehart, 1942.
33. Kaback, G. R. Vocational Personalities, an Application of the Rorschach Group Method. Contributions to Education, No. 924. New York: Bureau of Publications, Teachers College, Columbia University, 1946.
34. Kerr, W. A. "Labor Turnover and Its Correlates." Journal of Applied Psychology, XXXI (August, 1947), 366 - 371.
35. Kitson, H. D. "Creating Vocational Interests." Occupations, XX (May, 1942), 567 - 571.
36. Kornhauser, A. W. "The Technique of Measuring Employee Attitudes." Personnel, IX (February, 1933), 99 - 107.
37. -----. "Psychological Studies of Employee Attitudes." Journal of Consulting Psychology, VIII (May - June, 1944), 127 - 143.
38. Lewis, J. A. "Kuder Preference Record and MMPI Scores for Two Occupational Groups." Journal of Consulting Psychology, XI (July - August, 1947), 194 - 201.
39. Lorge, I. "The Prediction of Vocational Success." Personnel Journal, XII (December, 1933), 189 - 197.
40. -----. "Retests after Ten Years." Journal of Educational Psychology, XXV (February, 1934), 136 - 141.
41. Lurie, W. "The Concept of Occupational Adjustment." Educational Psychological Measurement, II (January, 1942), 3 - 14.
42. Noall, I. S. "Pharmacy as an Occupation." Occupations, XV (March, 1937), 521 - 527.
43. Paterson, D. G., and J. G. Darley. Men, Women and Jobs. Minneapolis: University of Minnesota Press, 1936.
44. Remmers, H. H., and N. L. Gage. The Abilities and Interests of Pharmacy Freshmen. Pharmaceutical Survey Monograph No. 1. Washington, D. C.: American Council on Education, 1948.
45. Ryan, T. A., and B. R. Johnson. "Interest Scores in the Selection of Salesmen and Servicemen: Occupational vs. Ability Group Scoring Keys." Journal of Applied Psychology, XXVI (August, 1942), 543 - 562.

46. Sarbin, T. R., and H. C. Anderson. "A Preliminary Study of the Relation of Measured Interest Patterns and Occupational Dissatisfaction." Educational Psychological Measurement, II (January, 1942), 23 - 26.
47. Seidman, J. M., and G. Watson. "Satisfaction in Work." Journal of Consulting Psychology, IV (July - August, 1940), 117 - 120.
48. Speer, G. S. "The Vocational Interests of Engineering and Non-Engineering Students." Journal of Psychology, XXV (April, 1948), 357 - 363.
49. Strong, E. K. Jr. "Procedure for Scoring an Interest Test." Psychological Clinic, XIX (April, 1930), 63 - 72.
50. -----. "Interests of Engineers." Personnel Journal, VII (April, 1929), 444 - 454.
51. -----. Change of Interests with Age. Stanford University: Stanford University Press, 1931.
52. -----. "Interest Maturity." Personnel Journal, XII (August, 1933), 77 - 90.
53. -----. "Selection of Students for Dental Colleges." Proceedings of the American Association of Dental Colleges, X, 121 - 133, 1933.
54. -----. "Aptitudes versus Attitudes in Vocational Guidance." Journal of Applied Psychology, XVIII (August, 1934), 501 - 515.
55. -----. "Classification of Occupations by Interests." Personnel Journal, XII (April, 1934), 301 - 313.
56. -----. "Interests and Sales Ability." Personnel Journal, XIII (December, 1934), 204 - 216.
57. -----. "Permanence of Vocational Interests." Journal of Educational Psychology, XXV (May, 1934), 336 - 344.
58. -----. "Relation of Interest to Ability in Terms of Life Insurance Interest Scores and Sales Production." Psychological Bulletin, XXXI (October 1934), 594.
59. -----. "The Vocational Interest Test." Occupations, XII (June, 1934), 49 - 56.
60. -----. "Predictive Value of the Vocational Interest Test." Journal of Educational Psychology, XXVI (May, 1935), 331 - 349.
61. -----. "Interests of Men and Women." Journal of Social Psychology, VII (February, 1936), 49 - 67.
62. -----. "Significance of the Point of Reference." Psychological Bulletin, XXXVI (July, 1939), 548.
63. -----. Vocational Interests of Men and Women. Stanford University: Stanford University Press, 1943.

BIBLIOGRAPHY

64. -----. *Manual for Vocational Interest Blank for Men.* Stanford University: Stanford University Press, 1945.
65. Strong, E. K., Jr., and H. MacKenzie. "Permanence of Interests of Adult Men." *Journal of Social Psychology,* I (February, 1930), 152 - 159.
66. Super, D. E. "Occupational Level and Job Satisfaction." *Journal of Applied Psychology,* XXIII (October, 1939), 547 - 564.
67. -----. *Avocational Interest Patterns.* Stanford University: Stanford University Press, 1940.
68. -----. "Avocations and Vocational Adjustment." *Character and Personality,* X (September, 1941), 51 - 61.
69. -----. "Strong's Vocational Interests of Men and Women, a Special Review." *Psychological Bulletin,* XLII (June, 1945), 359 - 370.
70. -----. "Vocational Interests and Vocational Choice: Present Knowledge and Future Research in Their Relationships." *Educational Psychological Measurement,* VII (Autumn, 1947), 375 - 383.
71. -----. *Appraising Vocational Fitness.* New York: Harper and Brothers; 1949.
72. Taft, R., and A. Mullins. "Who Quits and Why." *Personnel Journal,* XXIV (February, 1946), 300 - 307.
73. Thorndike, E. L. *Prediction of Vocational Success.* New York: Commonwealth Fund, 1934.
74. -----. "Workers Satisfaction: Likes and Dislikes of Young People for Their Jobs." *Occupations,* XIII (May, 1935), 704 - 706.
75. Tussing, L. "An Investigation of the Possibilities of Measuring Personality Traits with Strong Vocational Interest Blank." *Educational Psychological Measurement,* II (January, 1942), 59 - 74.
76. Walker, H. *Elementary Statistical Methods.* New York: Henry Holt and Co., 1943.
77. Watson, G., and J. M. Seidman. "Dissatisfaction in Work." *Journal of Social Psychology,* XVII (February, 1943), 93 - 97.
78. Wightwick, M. I. *Vocational Interest Patterns.* Contributions to Education, No. 900. New York: Bureau of Publications, Teachers College, Columbia University, 1945.
79. Williamson, E. G. "An Analysis of the Young-Estabrook Studiousness Scale." *Journal of Applied Psychology,* XXI (June, 1937), 260 - 264.

80. Wolfle, D. "Annual Report of the Executive Secretary: 1948." American Psychologist, III (November, 1948), 503 - 506.
81. Wrenn, C. G. "Vocational Satisfaction of Stanford Graduates." Personnel Journal, XIII (June, 1934), 21 - 24.
82. Findings and Recommendations of the Pharmaceutical Survey. Washington, D. C.: American Council on Education, 1948.
83. Handbook of Pharmacy Law, Rules and Information. Albany: University of the State of New York, 1948.

Index

Age and pharmacy satisfaction, 18-20, 24-25
American Council on Education, 7-8
Anderson, H. C., 5
Apothecary and business pharmacists, difference between, 57; inadequate differentiation, 64-65; apothecary pharmacists, 8-9; scores of, on pharmacy scales, 54-56; compared with business pharmacists on scales, 55-57
Apothecary vs. Business Pharmacists Scale, 9; weighting, 33; variation from usual construction procedure, 35; reliability, 40; stability of items, 41; interoccupational discriminating power of, 42-49; satisfied and dissatisfied, 49-53, intra-occupational discriminating power of, 49-57; apothecary and business, 54-57; weakness of, 57; interrelationship with other pharmacy scales, 58-60; intercorrelations, 58-59; inter-half-scale correlations, 60; correlated with satisfaction, 61; inadequacy of explained, 64-65

Ballard, C. W., vii
Benge, E. J., 18
Berman, I. R., 35
Bordin, E. S., 44, 64
Burnham, P. S., 34
Business pharmacists, 8-9; scores of, on pharmacy scales, 55-56; compared with apothecary pharmacists on scales, 55-57

Carter, H. D., 1, 2, 44
Characteristics of 50 most and 50 least satisfied, 23-28
Characteristics of satisfied and dissatisfied, 18-28; nondifferentiating, 18-20; age, 18-20; differentiating, 21-23
Characteristics of validation-group pharmacists, 39-40
Chemists Scale, scores of pharmacists on, 42-45; scores of apothecary and business satisfied pharmacists compared, 48-49; scores of satisfied and dissatisfied compared, 51-53
Clendenen, D. M., viii, 46
Copell, D. F., 18
Correlations, coefficient of reliability of pharmacy scales, 40, 60; inter-half-scale, 41, 60; of scores on pharmacy scales, 58-59; of interest scores and index of satisfaction, 61
Covering letter, 13, 71
Criterion group, recommendations for selection of, 69
Criterion in selection of weight-norm group, success, 2-3; job satisfaction, 2-3, 5-6; ability in an occupation, 6; specialty within occupation, 6

Darley, J. G., 1, 5, 35
Davison, J., viii
Davison, S., viii
Dentists Scale, scores of pharmacists on, 42-45; scores of apothecary and business satisfied pharmacists compared, 48-49; scores of satisfied and dissatisfied compared, 51-53
Dickson, W. J., 10
Differentiating characteristics, satisfied and dissatisfied, of criterion group, 21-23; of validation group, 40
Differentiation, apothecary and business pharmacists, 8-9; inadequate differentiation, 64-65
Differentiation of intra-occupational interests, of specialties, v; among engineering students, 6; of ability groups, 6; of satisfied and dissatisfied, 49-54; of apothecary and business, 54-57
Dissatisfaction, due to working conditions, 30; misplacement, 30; maladjustment, 30-31; origins of, 30-31
Dissatisfied pharmacists, of criterion group, 17-18; of validation group, 39-40; scores of on non-pharmacy scales compared with satisfied, 51-53

81

Elliott, E. C., vii
Engineering student interest scale, 6
Estes, S. G., 6, 7
Evaluation of pharmacy interest scales, 61-65
Experience in pharmacy, years of and pharmacy satisfaction, 18, 24-25

Fisher, R. A., 14
Fisher, V. E., 31
Fryer, D., 1, 35
Fuller, S. E., 10

Gage, N. L., 44
Gaies, A. A., viii
Garrett, H. E., 40

Habbe, S., 30
Hahn, M. E., 5
Hand, T., 10, 11
Hanna, J. V., 31
Hewitt, H. G., viii
Hoppock, R., vii; review of job satisfaction literature, 10; definition of job satisfaction, 11; study of teacher satisfaction, 11; Job Satisfaction Blank No. 1, 13; on measuring satisfaction, 17; study of age and satisfaction, 18
Horn, D., 6, 7
Hypotheses of the study, 5-9; tests of, 41-57

Interest inventories, development of, 1; validity of 1; construction of scale, 3-4
Interest scales, recommended research, 69
Interest scores, of criterion and validation groups compared, 42; of pharmacists on non-pharmacy scales, 42-44; of pharmacists on business and science occupational scales compared, 43-45; of pharmacists and non-pharmacists compared, 46-49
Interests, and change in satisfaction, 63-64; relation to satisfaction, needed research on, 69
Interoccupational differentiation, by an occupational ability-group scale, 6
Interoccupational discriminating power of the pharmacy scales, 42-49
Interrelationship of pharmacy interest scales, 58-60

Interviews, limitation of, in research, 11; of Utica pharmacists, 14-15
Intra-occupational discriminating power of the pharmacy scales, 49-57
Ivanhoe, R., viii

Job satisfaction, as related to interests, v; and primary interest pattern, 5; as criterion, 5-6; origin of, 10; defined, 10-11; method of measurement, 10-11; effectiveness as criterion and point of reference, 62-64; recommendations for use of in selecting criterion group, 69; relation to interests, needed research on, 69
Job Satisfaction Blank No. 1, vii, 11
Johnson, B. R., 6-7, 9, 63

Kaback, G. R., 44, 63
Kerr, W. A., 30
Kessler, H., viii
Kessler, T., viii
Kitson, H. D., vii
Kuder Preference Record, 5

Lemon, A. B., vii
Life Insurance Salesmen Scale, scores of pharmacists on, 42-45; scores of apothecary and business satisfied pharmacists compared, 48-49; scores of satisfied and dissatisfied compared, 51-53
Lorge, I., vii, 1

Materials used in getting data, 13
"Medical" interest of pharmacists discussed, 42, 44
Medical students, 42-49; scores of, on pharmacy scales and Physicians Scale compared, 46-49
Men-in-general group, 6
Mullins, A., 18

New Haven Druggists' Association, vii, 39
Newton, H. C., viii
Noall, I. S., 9
Norms of pharmacy interest scales, 36-38

O'Brien, F. J., vii
Occupation in pharmacy and pharmacy satisfaction, 18, 27-28
Odom, C., 10

INDEX

Office Workers Scale, scores of pharmacists on, 42-45; scores of apothecary and business satisfied pharmacists compared, 48-49; scores of satisfied and dissatisfied compared, 51-53

Paterson, D. G., 35
Pharmacist, definition of, 9; qualities for success, 9
Pharmacists, sample of, percentage of returns, 15; percentage of satisfaction compared, earlier and later returns, 16; percentage of satisfaction compared, total sample and Utica subsample, 16; possible bias, 16; characteristics, 16; urban-rural distribution, 16; differentiation of satisfied and dissatisfied, 17; non-differentiating characteristics of satisfied and dissatisfied, 18-20; differentiating characteristics, 21-23; validation group, 39-40; criterion and validation groups compared, 39-40
Pharmacists, satisfied, 11-13; dissatisfied, 11-13; scores on non-pharmacy scales, 42-44; scores on business and science occupational scales compared, 43-45; interest in medicine, 44; scores of, compared with those of medical students, 46-49; differentiated by scales, 49-57; satisfied and dissatisfied, 49-53; apothecary and business, 54-57; scores of satisfied and dissatisfied on non-pharmacy scales compared, 51-53; apothecary and business, difference between, 57; interests and satisfaction of, correlated, 61; apothecary and business, inadequate differentiation, 64-65
Pharmacy interest scales, construction of, 32-38; weighting, 32-33; stability of weight, 33-34; variations from usual procedures of construction, 34-35; size of criterion groups, 35-36; composition of, 36; norms, 36-38; scores and letter grades, 37; distribution of grades and scores compared, 38; coefficients of reliability, 40, 60; stability of items, 41; inter-half-scale correlations, 41, 60; interoccupational discriminating power, 42-49; intercorrelation of scores, 58-59; correlation with satisfaction index, 61; interrelationship, 58-61; evaluation, 61-65
Pharmacy organization, nature of, and pharmacy satisfaction, 21, 27, 40
Pharmacy profession, reason for use in study, 7; tests for selection of students, 8
Pharmacy satisfaction, correlated with pharmacy interest scores, 61; effectiveness as point of reference, 62-63; stability of, 63-64
Pharmacy Satisfaction Scale, 13, 72-73; method of scoring, 17; "sorry" responses, 17-18
Physicians Scale, scores of pharmacists on, 42-45; scores of medical students on, 46-48; scores of apothecary and business satisfied pharmacists compared, 48-49; scores of satisfied and dissatisfied compared, 51-53
Point of reference, 3-4; business pharmacists, 4; dissatisfied, 4; men in general, 4, 6; dissatisfied, 6; inferior workers, 6; subgroup of engineer students, 6-7; effectiveness of satisfaction as, 62-63; recommended research on, 69
Prescription work, percentage of, and pharmacy satisfaction, 21-23, 26-27, 40

Questionnaire returns, methods of increasing, 14

Reasons for dissatisfaction, 28-31; hours of work, 28-29; "ethical" pharmacy, 29; earnings, 29-30
Recommendations for further research, 69
Relatives in pharmacy and pharmacy satisfaction, 18, 24
Reliability of scores, 40
Remmers, H. H., viii, 44
Research, recommendations for, 69
Robinson, H. A., 10
Ryan, T. A., 6-7, 9, 63

Sales Managers Scale, scores of pharmacists on, 42-45; scores of apothecary and business satisfied pharmacists compared, 48-49; scores of satisfied and dissatisfied compared, 51-53

INDEX

Sample of pharmacists see Pharmacists, sample of

Sarbin, T. R., 5

Satisfaction of pharmacists, 17-28; and age, 18-20, 24-25; and occupation in pharmacy, 18, 27-28; and relatives in pharmacy, 18, 24; and urban-rural status, 18, 24; and World War II veteran status, 18, 24; and years of experience, 18, 24-25; and percentage of prescription work, 21-23, 26-27, 40; and nature of organization, 21, 27, 40

Satisfied pharmacists, of criterion group, 18-31; of validation group, 39-40; scores of on non-pharmacy scales compared with dissatisfied, 51-53

Satisfied vs. Dissatisfied Pharmacists Scale, weighting, 33; variation from usual construction procedure, 35; reliability, 40; stability of items, 41; interoccupational discriminating power of, 42-49; satisfied and dissatisfied, 49-53; intra-occupational discriminating power of, 49-57; apothecary and business, 54-57; interrelationship with other pharmacy scales, 58-60; intercorrelations, 58-59; inter-half-scale correlations, 60; correlated with satisfaction, 61

Scoring, Vocational Interest Scale for Pharmacists, vii

Seidman, J. M., 29

Shaffer, L. F., vii

Shaffer, R. H., 10

Size of criterion groups, 35-36

Spiegler, S., 10

Stability of items, 41

Stability of pharmacy satisfaction, 63-64; and change of interests, 63-64

Stability of weights, 33-34

Strong, E. K. Jr., vii; study of life insurance salesman, 1; study of Stanford University seniors, 1; on differentiation of interests, 3; on interests as predictors of satisfaction, 3; description of his Vocational Interest Blank for Men, 13; on stability of weights, 34; on size of criterion group, 35; on change of interests, 44, 64

Strong's Vocational Interest Blank. see Vocational Interest Blank for Men

Subjects of the study, 14-15; method of selection, 14

Summary of study, 66-68; findings, 68

Super, D. E., Foreword, vii; on interests as predictors of satisfaction, 3; on satisfaction, 3; on maladjustment and dissatisfaction, 10; study of age and satisfaction, 18-20; on change of interests, 44, 64

Taft, R., 18

Thorndike, E. L., 1

Urban-rural status and pharmacy satisfaction, 18, 24

Utica pharmacists, viii, 14-15

Utica Pharmacy Association, 15

Validation group of pharmacists, 39-40; compared with criterion group, 39-40

Veteran status, of World War II, and pharmacy satisfaction, 18, 24

Vocational Interest Blank for Men, 1-2, 13

Vocational Interest Scale for Pharmacists, variation from usual construction procedure, 34-35; reliability, 40; stability of items, 41; interoccupational discriminating power of, 42-49; satisfied and dissatisfied, 49-53; intra-occupational discriminating power of, 49-57; apothecary and business, 54-57; interrelationship with other pharmacy scales, 58-60; intercorrelations, 58-59; inter-half-scale correlations, 60; correlated with satisfaction, 61

Vocational interests, change of, discussed, 44

Vocational interest scales, establishing weights, 7

Watson, G., 29

Weighting items, procedure of, 32-33

Williams, C. I., 5

Wimmer, C. A., vii

Wolfle, D., 1

Yates, F., 14

Zlatchin, P., 10

Bei Fragen zur Produktsicherheit wenden Sie sich bitte an:
If you have any questions regarding product safety,
please contact:

Walter de Gruyter GmbH
Genthiner Straße 13
10785 Berlin
productsafety@degruyterbrill.com